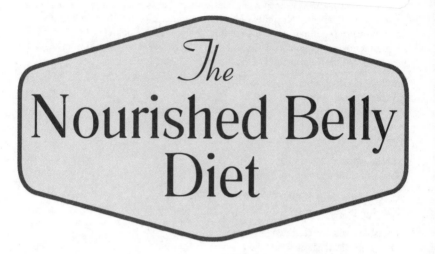

# The Nourished Belly Diet

21-Day Plan to Heal Your Gut,
Kick-Start Weight Loss, Boost Energy
and Have You Feeling Great

Tammy Chang

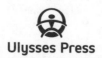

Ulysses Press

Published in the US by:
Ulysses Press
P.O. Box 3440
Berkeley, CA 94703
www.ulyssespress.com

ISBN13: 978-1-61243-550-3
Library of Congress Control Number: 2015952134

Printed in the United States by United Graphics Inc.
10 9 8 7 6 5 4 3 2 1

Acquisitions Editor: Casie Vogel
Managing Editor: Claire Chun
Editor: Renee Rutledge
Proofreader: Lauren Harrison
Index: Sayre Van Young
Front cover design: what!design @ whatweb.com
Interior design and layout: what!design @ whatweb.com
Cover artwork: fruits/vegetables © Kateryna Sednieva/shutterstock.com; label © Kovacs Tamas/shutterstock.com
Interior illustrations: pages 31 and 54 © Sarah Trent

Distributed by Publishers Group West

NOTE TO READERS: This book has been written and published strictly for informational and educational purposes only. It is not intended to serve as medical advice or to be any form of medical treatment. You should always consult your physician before altering or changing any aspect of your medical treatment and/or undertaking a diet regimen, including the guidelines as described in this book. Do not stop or change any prescription medications without the guidance and advice of your physician. Any use of the information in this book is made on the reader's good judgment after consulting with his or her physician and is the reader's sole responsibility. This book is not intended to diagnose or treat any medical condition and is not a substitute for a physician.

To my family and friends

# Contents

## CHAPTER 7
## Holistic Nutrition 101 ..............................179

# Introduction

Welcome! The fact that you've picked up this book means that you are interested in something new for your health. *Yes!* Whether you are just starting on the journey or you've been on this path for a while, I'm excited that you are here. Each of us is here for different reasons: maybe you want to lose a few pounds, crave more energy, or just need some inspiration in the kitchen. Our common connection is a target of optimum health. I have my own evolving target, and every day is a practice for me to get as close as possible. Today, writing this book is a wonderful reminder of what I'm working on.

This book is my opportunity to share what I've learned throughout my life from various teachers, self-directed study, dear friends, and of course my clients! With loving guidance and experimentation, I discovered that pretty much everything I wanted to change about my health can be transformed by how I eat.

*The Nourished Belly Diet* is a 21-day guide to what I've discovered; it consists of 21 days of eating whole, traditional foods. There are different levels of participation, and if you are open to following it, I have a strong feeling you will see a shift in your health and body. Eating in this way has stabilized my weight, cleared my break-out-prone skin, and made me feel strong and grounded. This is not about being perfect; it's about knowing how to come to a way of eating that can bring you back into balance.

I'm so thankful that I've come to where I am because before, my mind-set about food was very toxic. When I was a child, I spent a lot of time trying to be what others thought I should be. I played instruments from a young age, competed in sports, and studied hard in school. I was a "good" kid, and I felt successful in many of these areas. However, there was one area that I felt like a failure—I was a chubby child.

Society treats people who have extra weight on them horribly. Instead of seeing a *person*, the tendency is to judge people on their weight and make assumptions about their self-control or general health. (In reality, many different shapes and sizes can be healthy. Plus, it's about finding and maintaining the size where you *feel* your best, not where society tells you to be.)

By the time I reached high school, I had an obsession with my body and what I ate. I regarded my body and my eating addictions as the enemy. I was either doing something "bad" and eating something bad, or I was being "good" and eating something good. I would compare myself to my girlfriends and wish that I had their body or that I could wear bikinis without feeling self-conscious.

I tried as hard as I could to follow the conventional wisdom at the time, which was to eat low-fat foods, carb load before swim meets, and exercise exercise exercise. I was a competitive swimmer from a young age, and if you know anything about swim teams, it's that they practice...a *lot*. We had morning practices before school and two-hour practices after school. I simply thought that I would burn off anything I ate, so I ate no-fat ice cream and peanut butter before practices, thinking hey, I was going to work it off!

Whatever I was doing was detrimental. My weight fluctuated back and forth, my sugar intake was insane, and I didn't feel in control of my eating. Most importantly, I didn't feel good about myself. Truly loving the body that we are given is not a common thing. People often feel the need to have better hips, a smaller gut, less jiggly arms...it doesn't end!

In my twenties, I was in the middle of living one of the worst, most stressful years of my life. Having just moved to New York City, I was an inexperienced, first-year teacher in a "hard to staff" school in Brownsville, Brooklyn.

Luckily, this was also the time I discovered a way of moving that I loved: capoeira (a Brazilian martial art that has now become a large part of my life). Through class, I met a holistic health coach named Molly. The first time I heard about what Molly did (oh, you counsel people on what they should be eating?), my first impression was surprise that this was actually a *thing*. As the year went on and I realized how out of control I felt, I decided that maybe this was something I needed. I began seeing her as a client, and in hindsight, to have someone hold the space for me to examine my life when the outside was so utterly chaotic was a blessing.

Working with a health coach set me on a path of learning how to cook for myself, experimenting with different foods that I had never eaten before (what is this quinoa?), and getting hip to the fact that food and mood are connected.

Most importantly, I began to look at food in a different way. Instead of always seeing food as something to control, I started to see food as healthful and nourishing. When I made a meal for myself and others, I felt a sense of accomplishment. I saw that making meals together was a wonderful way to connect with people—and real food tastes amazing!

This set me on a voracious path reading every possible book on nutrition. I moved to North Carolina and life slowed down enough for me to experiment in the kitchen. I made an effort to buy high-quality produce from the farmers markets.

One day, I decided that I had had enough of the public school system, and I decided to take a road trip with a couple of girlfriends across the country; this turned into my springboard for deep discovery about good food. I've cooked and shared many wonderful meals since I left North Carolina and found my way to California. I have harvested and eaten myself silly with peaches and snap peas and apples as I worked on an organic farm and did little experiments with my health as I went through holistic nutrition school at Bauman College in Berkeley.

Throughout all of this, my body image issues still surface (being overly critical), but it's overpowered by a love of food. I love food. I love seeing food grown, I love picking it, I love cooking it, I love sharing it. And all those things that I used to care about have resolved themselves. My weight is stable, I've cultivated a movement practice that keeps me strong, and my skin, which always gave me anxiety, is clear and smooth.

I'm now in my late thirties, and although I don't know everything, I have experimented enough with food to find out there is not only ONE way to eat. Even though this book has the word "diet" in the title, let's look at a diet as *a way to eat*. Not the way that I used to look at the word, which meant restriction, counting calories, and being "good." In my life and with my clients, I have found these things to backfire. It pits food against us, which is not its role at all. Food nourishes us. It energizes us. It is a way to love, not only ourselves, but others. So let me share with you what I've learned about nourishing our bellies and souls with *The Nourished Belly Diet*.

With love,

Tammy

# Why the Nourished Belly Diet?

There is very little doubt that the country is in the midst of a health crisis. We are spending trillions on health care,[1] one in three adult Americans are currently considered obese,[2] and one in three Americans are expected to develop diabetes by 2050.[3] Something needs to change.

We've come a long way in disease prevention; as a society, we've figured out how to treat water, produce food in a sanitary and safe way, and deal with waste treatment. In trauma care, we are able to save lives. People are without a doubt living longer.

---

1   Munro, Dan. "Annual US Healthcare Spending Hits $3.8 Trillion." *Forbes.* February 2, 2014, http://www.forbes.com/sites/danmunro/2014/02/02/annual-u-s-healthcare-spending-hits-3-8-trillion/.

2   "Adult Obesity Facts," Centers for Disease Control and Prevention, last modified June 16, 2015, accessed September 15, 2015, http://www.cdc.gov/obesity/data/adult.html.

3   Boyle, James P., Theodore Thompson, Edward W. Gregg, Lawrence E. Barker, and David F. Williamson. "Projection of the Year 2050 Burden of Diabetes in the US Adult Population: Dynamic Modeling of Incidence, Mortality, and Prediabetes Prevalence." *Population Health Metrics.* October 22, 2010, http://www.ncbi.nlm.nih.gov/pubmed/20969750.

But what about healthier? What about quality of life, community, and interconnectedness? What about growing old while still being able to enjoy the sunshine, travel, and play with grandkids? I have a mission to move my body and enjoy my life until the very end, and in order to do that, I need to take care of this body I've been given.

I think we can all agree that the obesity epidemic, the amount of hours we are conditioned to work, and the increase in degenerative diseases, such as diabetes, Parkinson's disease, and Alzheimer's, have all limited the ability to enjoy life to the fullest in our twilight years.

There is the argument that we are living longer, so of course different diseases will plague us. It's true. From a biological standpoint, we weren't necessarily meant to live to old age. We were meant to reproduce. However, we humans are a particularly crafty bunch and have found ways through science and technology to multiply extremely rapidly and to live longer and longer.

Let's use all that we've learned about the human body to live in a way that promotes longevity and joy, where we *use* all of this scientific knowledge to our advantage. What's one extremely important way? We need nutrients! (To find out exactly which nutrients we need, check out Chapter 7 for a Holistic Nutrition 101 Tutorial.)

Physiological processes need nutrients to happen. It's biology. However, we need to be cautious, because it never boils down to just one. Just because you *hear* that a certain nutrient can protect against cancer does not mean that you should rush out and take it every day. We need *all* of them. For example, nutrients come in and out of the cell most efficiently with the right ratio of sodium to potassium.[4] The right amount of calcium in the blood is crucial for our muscles to relax.[5] Zinc and vitamin A work together for

4   Kamen, Betty, and Paul Kamen. *Everything You Always Wanted to Know about Potassium but Were Too Tired to Ask: How Potassium Affects High Blood Pressure, Fatigue, the Aging Process, Alcoholism, Headaches and More.* Novata, CA: Nutrition Encounter, 1992.

5   Ibid, 15.

our eyesight to function correctly.[6] These are just a few examples of how many nutrients work together to make the exquisite body run the way it does.

We also have the added pressure to consume all these different nutrients in different amounts, since many of them compete for absorption. Plus, certain nutrients need certain mediums to be absorbed, like fat is essential for vitamins A, D, and E to be absorbed. How can we keep all these varying conditions straight, especially how many milligrams of what vitamin to take and when, and with what?

Nature, however, has made the answer simple for us: Just eat whole foods! I like to call them regenerative foods because they help the body to regenerate many times over the course of a lifetime. Each cell in the body has varying lifespans. Stomach cells renew themselves every three to four days, skin cells live about three weeks, and red blood cells three months.[7]

In order to regenerate and to function optimally, we need nutrients. Plain and simple.

Our bodies run the way they do because of how we choose to live. Eating is one of the most fundamental ways to ensure we live long, mobile, healthy lives. Food is incorporated into our cells. It is necessary for our brains to make connections and our hearts to continue to beat without conscious thought.

# Bringing True Eating Back

These days, there are so many fad diets, supplement powders, and meal replacements, not to mention juicing! So many people ask me which protein powder to buy or which juice cleanse is the most beneficial. What I wish people would ask me is: What foods

6   "Micronutrient Information Center" *Zinc*, Linus Pauling Center. Accessed September 15, 2015, http://lpi.oregonstate.edu/mic/minerals/zinc.

7   Radford, Benjamin. "Does the Human Body Really Replace Itself Every 7 Years?" *LiveScience*, April 4, 2011, http://www.livescience.com/33179-does-human-body-replace-cells-seven-years.html.

should I be eating? This question not only makes more sense, but it makes feeding ourselves a lot more enjoyable. I can't remember a powder tasting all that good, but give me a freshly picked tomato ripened on the vine? Yum. Eating and enjoying our food is what we should be getting back to, not fad diets, fasting, or cleansing! *The Nourished Belly Diet* is all about bringing real food back to the table and to our lives.

# Getting Back in the Kitchen

Many people don't want the hassle of making their own food, and I get it. Our lives can be crazy; with kids, jobs, and social schedules, all of us are guilty of putting off what we've come to see as the "chore" of cooking. Dealing with dishes can be too much to handle on those crazy days.

However, I've found that those who take on learning how to be skilled in the kitchen become the key holders to their own health. Talk about empowerment! Cooking is a skill, like playing the violin, and as with any skill, practice creates efficiency and allows for creativity. Lucky for us, there are just a few fundamentals to learn, and once we have that, we are free to feed ourselves with abandon!

I was especially heartened about getting back into the kitchen after I read Michael Pollan's book *Cooked,* many points of which are also in a 2009 *New York Times* article, "Out of the Kitchen, Onto the Couch."[8] Pollan gives the unsettling statistic that the average person spends 27 minutes a *day* on food prep and four minutes cleaning up. Dividing that amount by three meals per day equates to nine minutes prepping each meal. I don't think I have to tell you what nutrients and quality we sacrifice for convenience.

Pollan also explains that although we spend less time making food, we are eating more of it. Since 1977, we've added half a

---

8   Pollan, Michael. "Out of the Kitchen, Onto the Couch." *The New York Times*, August 1, 2009, http://www.nytimes.com/2009/08/16/magazine/16letters-t-OUTOFTHEKITC_LETTERS.html.

meal to our daily food intake. Cooking less is also correlated with obesity rates, as well as being a better predictor of health than social class.

Cooking *matters* in terms of health. I always start to feel bloated and brain foggy when I eat out too often. I feel it most when I'm on vacation and I don't have much choice in the matter. Restaurants use a lot more salt than I do at home, and who knows what types of oils they are using.

Plus, cooking is a beautiful skill. It's a wonderful blend of chemistry and art. There's a little science nerd in me that loves to learn about what substances in foods bring out flavors and the interactions of cells with cold or hot. It's an endless form of learning. I loved reading Harold McGee's *On Food and Cooking,* and *Cook's Illustrated,* a magazine that doesn't necessarily let nutrition guide its ingredients, but provides a scientific lens on experimentation with recipes. For example, it's from reading these types of resources that I learned exactly what baking powder and baking soda do to baked goods. (They are both leavening agents; baking soda leavens with the help of an acid, so your recipe usually has an acid, like lemon juice or chocolate, and baking powder is made up of baking soda plus an acid, usually cream of tartar. Did I just blow your mind? )

So getting back to the kitchen is important. But we are still super busy, right? How do we fit it all in? A little organization (an important piece of the Nourished Belly Diet) is immeasurably helpful. Most of the recipes in this book are perfect for batch cooking, and figuring out a schedule for shopping and cooking make getting back into the kitchen manageable and routine.

Having a hand in the food that we eat goes an extremely long way toward feeling healthier. We have control over sourcing, control over choosing the right kinds of fats, and the very act of cooking gets our systems ready for digestion. When we see food and smell the wonderful smells of the kitchen, it stimulates our vagus nerve, which primes our body to eat and digest. Getting back into the kitchen is just part of the Nourished Belly Diet process. All we need to do is learn things one dish at a time.

## Supporting Local Farmers

Most of us don't grow our own food, and if you are, that's great! With the population growing, however, supply is an important thing to think about. One cultural phenomenon that I love is the push to support local businesses. Oakland, California, does a great job with this, and even during my last trip home to Toledo, Ohio, I found magazines dedicated to keeping our money in the community. When we support small, local businesses, a greater percentage of the money we spend will stay in the community as opposed to lining the pockets of some faraway investors.

This is especially important when it comes to our food. When we support local growers, we support a particular way of living that is better for the environment and an occupation that has been slowly dying off: farming. Less than 2 percent of Americans are farmers, with the average age of farmers in 2012 being 58.3 years old.[9] With our population steadily increasing, supply is increasingly important.

It's no wonder why fewer young people are entering into the profession: The normal average cost for a family farm is $109,359 per farm per year.[10] Yet, 75 percent of farms make $50,000 a year or less.[11] This is a pretty big discrepancy.

One of my favorite experiences in my food journey was working on a farm for five months on the central coast of California. It is another life entirely to live almost completely off the land. We had a full home garden that had everything you could want—an

9   Ibid.

10  "Demographics," EPA, last modified April 14, 2013, accessed September 15, 2015, http://www.agcensus.usda.gov/Publications/2012/Preliminary_Report/Highlights.pdf.

11  "Preliminary Report Highlights; US Farms and Farmers," February 1, 2014, accessed September 15, 2015, http://www.agcensus.usda.gov/Publications/2012/Preliminary_Report/Highlights.pdf.

orchard full of peaches, apples, and pears, chickens for eggs, and we raised chickens for slaughter.

As idyllic as this sounds, farming is a lot of work. Animals need daily care, and vegetables and orchards need planting, nurturing, weeding, fertilizing, harvesting, and packaging. It seems a steal to pay just a few dollars for something that took so much work to grow.

I love that there are farmers out there who are passionate about the food they produce. As a society, we need to encourage this, because unfortunately, if everyone in this country wanted to start eating organic and only buying pasture-raised meats, the supply isn't there. Not enough people out there are growing food in a sustainable, organic way. Underlying the Nourished Belly Diet is knowing where your food dollars are going. Sometimes our hands are tied, but I really do love when my food dollars go to support a farmer directly, or I shop at a small, family-owned grocery store or eat at locally owned restaurants.

Start by making an effort to find a farmers market close to you. Or, seek out a local restaurant where you might enjoy eating. Everything you do is a small step in the larger journey.

# Saving Money

Money influences all of us, one way or another. I definitely pay attention to where the best deals are and have in my head which stores and markets I'll buy certain things from. Eating healthy, for me, is a priority, and if I were going to spend money on anything, it's good food. (I also like soft, organic sheets because we spend a *lot* of time sleeping.)

Most people don't always have this as a priority, but to me things seem a bit skewed. "Organic food is too expensive," I often hear, even from my own parents. They almost had a heart attack when they heard that the pastured eggs I buy cost $8. However, most people don't bat an eye at spending $4.65 for a White Chocolate

Mocha at Starbucks or buying a $6 to $12 cocktail. That's *one* drink that will keep you occupied for maybe an hour? Eggs I'll eat the entire week!

What makes a gigantic dent in your pocket is eating out. Some may argue that there are cheap places to eat, but cheap food usually means low quality. Plus, you will most likely pay down the line in health care costs! When you eat at home, you can buy good, quality foods and save that money for your next vacation. You do need to commit to spending extra money on high-quality, organic, or pasture-raised products. Commercial food has been artificially kept cheap through farm subsidies, and quality is not as high. Honestly, I would rather pay $20 for an extremely nourishing whole chicken that could feed me for days *and* give me bone broth than $20 at a regular dinner out.

Let's look at some numbers for one person during an average work week: five days. Let's eat breakfast at home, and lowball the amount for coffee to go and lunch and dinner out.

Coffee break: $2
Lunch: $10
Dinner: $15
**Total per day: $27**
**Total per work week: $135**

Now let's take a look at how things add up with the Nourished Belly Diet, when you are buying local, organic, and pastured products.

Eggs: $8
Meats: $40
Grains: $5
Veggies: $25
Fruits: $10
Snacks: $20
**Total per work week: $108**

I eat out occasionally, and I do so with gusto. I love sharing meals with friends, and indulging once in a while. But on the whole, I prefer to make my own meals because I *know* that I will feel better doing so, and my wallet will thank me. You will too, trust me.

As we go further along in the book, we'll talk more about all the different components of completely nourishing ourselves, plus the first steps that can get you started.

# The Nourished Soul and Body

The Nourished Belly Diet mainly looks at food, but it can't just be about food. Health is not just one thing. It's the way you live your life: what you do with your days, the stress that plagues you, and what is in your physical environment. It's not possible to tackle all of these things at once, and if you are reading this book, you are probably pretty motivated to work on improving your health through nutrition (awesome!). Life change is about doing things one small step at a time, ideally in a community of like-minded people and sharing what you are doing all the way.

## The Nourished Belly Philosophy

| Nourishing the Soul | Nourishing the Body |
| --- | --- |
| Self-Love | Movement |
| Life Work | Sleep |
| Feeding the Mind | Environment |
| Managing Stress | Hydration |
| Community | Nourishing Foods |

# Nourishing the Soul

Another way of saying nourishing the soul is practicing self-love. When you take the time out of your day to cook for yourself or make a meal for your family, it's a way that you show yourself and others love. In Ayurveda, a traditional Hindu system of medicine, you impart love into the food that you make. (An argument could therefore be made that when you are in a crabby mood you impart this energy into the food as well.)

Much of the work that I do with clients deals with the idea of self-care. Many times, we get wrapped up in working and doing the best job we can for others that we forget about ourselves. If you don't take care of yourself, you can't adequately take care of others. No one can put you first except you! I know that if I'm not adequately rested or fed, I start to feel bitter. Thoughts go through my head like "why isn't anyone helping me?" or "why do I have to do everything myself?" If I'm taking care of myself, however, the work I do for others is a joy and a privilege.

I ask all my clients what they do for self-care, and many of them do not have an answer. As with everything, starting small is key. You can start soaking your feet in hot water, taking a bath, getting a massage, or doing a three-minute meditation. Treating yourself is completely worth it because you are invaluable...really! Only one you exists in this entire world!

All of the following ideas are different ways to practice self-love.

# Life Work

You can have the best nutrition in the world and be eating all the right things, but if you aren't living a life that you love, then what's the point? All of us have different paths. Maybe you were born to be a parent and caregiver, perhaps you were meant to share your gifts through playing music or saving the world through technology. What is it that calls to you?

I have always believed in following my heart, and I've really found my calling in teaching about nutrition, holistic health, and movement. At times it definitely hasn't been easy: going against convention (Asian parents!), not having financial security, working always for the next project. However, it has always been fulfilling and thus, joyful. Pursuing my passion also keeps me motivated to live in a way that supports my health so that I feel good physically to keep motivated and moving forward.

Jobs can sometimes be a means to an end, and there are many people who enjoy jobs and also follow their passions on the side. Among my clients and vast networks, however, unhappiness with work is one of the top reasons for feeling discontent.

I recently examined *why* I do anything. Why I love learning and teaching about nutrition and movement. I have boiled down my *why* to one statement: Whether it be through food, discovering what they love to do, or moving their bodies, people I touch *will* be more joyful. Somehow.

What's your why? Why do you do the things you do? You alone can make up the answer to this, so get creative! I loved reading the book *The War of Art* by Steven Pressfield because he talks about the value of being creative, which I take to mean creating something for the world. He says, "It's a gift to the world and every being in it. Don't cheat us of your contribution. Give us what you've got."[12]

Another path to thinking about your *why* is to make a list of things that you value, and then compare them with what you do. Are they in alignment? If yes, great, and if no, then that's great feedback!

## Feeding the Mind

How engaged are you in following your curiosity?

When I was teaching elementary school, one of my goals as a teacher was to create inspired learners in my classroom. I hated all the testing that public school kids go through because I would rather make more time for kids to chase their curiosity. I firmly believe that to stay motivated and excited about life, we have to keep learning. I'm always inspired when I hear that someone is following an interest and deepening their knowledge. Especially when I hear people talk about what they love!

You can engage your curiosity in little ways every day, such as reading an article or asking a friend to explain something. I always like to look back through my day and ask myself, "What did I learn today?" Hopefully, this process and this book will guide you to learn a few things!

## Managing Stress

Stress is one of the few very well-researched triggers of poor health. What I want to keep reiterating in this section is that it won't matter if you eat the best diet in the world, if you are chronically stressed, you will deplete yourself and eventually create the perfect storm for disease.

Robert Sapolsky has a wonderful book on this called *Why Zebras Don't Get Ulcers*, and he explains that there are two modes that the body functions in, the parasympathetic and sympathetic.[13]

---

12  Pressfield, Steven. *The War of Art: Break Through the Blocks and Win Your Inner Creative Battles.* New York: Black Irish Entertainment, 2012.

13  Sapolsky, Robert M. *Why Zebras Don't Get Ulcers: The Acclaimed Guide to Stress, Stress-Related Diseases, and Coping.* New York: W.H. Freeman and Company, 1998.

The sympathetic mode is called our fight-or-flight mode, where we are getting ready to run from that tiger. In this mode, all of our nonessential systems turn off, including our digestive system, immune system, and reproductive system. Our bodies need to conserve maximum energy to run for our lives.

The problem with daily life is when we can't distinguish between running from a tiger or rushing to get the kids out the door to school and then rush to work, or perhaps the deadline that is a few weeks away. This is what Sapolsky brings attention to as chronic stress.

If you think about all of these important systems shutting off—digestion, immunity, reproduction—doesn't it make sense that we get sick easily when we are stressed? And that our food just seems to sit in our bellies sometimes?

So now what? We can't just snap our fingers and make our responsibilities go away. But things like meditation, gratitude practices, and exercise are now being thoroughly researched and are shown to work! They can sound super hippie dippie, I know, but these practices make a big difference in people's lives, and what's the harm in trying? There are many meditation centers sprouting up in communities and yoga centers. Even apps exist that can get you started!

## Community

This is the last piece I want to touch on in this section because community is so vital to nourishment. In his book *The Story of the Human Body: Evolution, Health, and Disease*, Daniel Lieberman posits that part of why we evolved to our current state is because of our enhanced ability to cooperate and work together. He states, "Humans are unusually good at working together, we share food and other crucial resources, we help raise one another's children, we pass on useful information, and we even sometimes risk our lives to aid friends or even strangers in need."[14]

---

14  Lieberman, Daniel. *The Story of the Human Body: Evolution, Health, and Disease.* New York: Pantheon, 2013. Kindle edition.

A sense of belonging is a theme that runs through many philosophies of health and mental well-being. Community and support systems are at the top of my value lists. The times that I notice I'm most sad is when a feeling of isolation creeps into my mind. I think, ultimately, this is a feeling we all have, and when I can tap into feeling connected, whether it be through meditation or through connecting with my family or friends, the world is a completely different place.

Ask yourself if you are happy with the communities that surround you. If yes, then how can you deepen those relationships, and if not, who is the type of person you want to connect with, and where could you find them?

# Nourishing the Body

We are almost to talking about what to put in our mouths, almost! There's just a few things that I think are really important that go along with nourishing our bodies. The idea of holistic health is incomplete when you just focus on just *one* of any of these areas. Again, it's great to focus on them one at a time to incorporate them into your life, but it's the entire picture that we are working toward.

## Movement

Oh, movement! This is my other true love and joy—if I don't move my body every day, I feel it. There are so many ways to move that feel oh so good—stretching, using your muscles to lift weights, working out your breath and heart with aerobic activity. When you start to move in a way you like, you start to see that it just feels really good. Plus, your body was *made* to move. As you start to learn more about the human body, it's a shame *not* to use it.

When it comes to staying trim, exercise alone will not lead to weight loss. You can't just work off a bad diet. In tandem with exercise, feeding yourself the right foods to help your metabolism work efficiently and effectively is required if you are looking to maintain a certain weight. Besides weight, however, exercise is crucial to maintaining the body that you were given so that you can have an active quality of life.

I've seen bodies stop moving because of lack of movement. It is an unfortunate thing when the mind wants to move, but the body cannot respond. Daily movement is really the simple remedy to being able to *use* the body throughout your lifetime.

If you think of your body as the way you experience the world, then it just makes sense to keep it moving. Don't just listen to me, however—many experts have said the same thing. Some benefits to movement:

- Releases endorphins to improve mood
- Allows for lymphatic drainage
- Increases synovial fluid in joints (and therefore lubrication and nourishment)
- Keeps body flexible and strong
- Enhances quality of sleep
- Increases energy

You know that exercise is necessary, but how do you incorporate it into your life? According to the Office of Disease Prevention, "adults should do at least 150 minutes (2 hours and 30 minutes) a week of moderate-intensity, or 75 minutes (1 hour and 15 minutes) a week of vigorous-intensity aerobic physical activity, or an equivalent combination of moderate- and vigorous-intensity aerobic activity. Aerobic activity should be performed in episodes of at least 10 minutes, and preferably, it should be spread throughout the week."[15]

While I think guidelines like this can be helpful, I also think this puts exercise, like calorie counting, into something that we try to measure instead of a way we try to live.

---

15  "Physical Activity Guidelines, Chapter 4: Active Adults," Office of Disease Prevention and Health Promotion, accessed September 15, 2015, http://health.gov/paguidelines/guidelines/chapter4.aspx.

I have always hated exercising for exercise's sake. When I was a teenager and really obsessed about calorie counting, I remember going to the gym and not leaving until I had burned 500 calories. What an un-fun way to exercise.

It's important to find something that you love to do to make it sustainable. Find friends to go on walks with, go to different classes and see what fits and what doesn't. I love taking classes, and I always know a class that's a good fit when I don't look at the clock to see how much time is left. Plus, many types of movement have great communities, so it's just about finding the right one, but there are so many out there: yoga, kickball, softball, soccer, capoeira (hint hint), salsa, circus, dance. There is something out there for everyone.

## Sleep

We spend a lot of our lives sleeping. We've been conditioned to think that sleeping is a waste of time, but it's anything but. Lack of sleep is an enormous stress on the body, and there are whole centers devoted to aiding people who chase the elusive good night's rest. According to the Institute of Medicine, in 2006, 50 to 70 million US adults suffered from sleep disorders.[16] This can be dangerous when linked to car crashes and work accidents.

Aside from possibly being lethal, insufficient sleep can seriously mess with your health. It can mess with memory, hormones, and cause weight gain. Yikes! Let's look into this a bit more.

According to the National Sleep Foundation, sleep is governed by two different processes.[17] The first is called the sleep/wake homeostasis. After you've been awake for a long time, your body will tell you that you need to sleep. The second is the light and dark cycles of the day, also called circadian rhythm. When your body perceives it's light out, it releases cortisol that helps you to

---

16 "Sleep Disorders and Sleep Deprivation: An Unmet Public Health Problem," Institute of Medicine, last modified March 26, 2006, accessed September 15, 2015, http://www.nap.edu/read/11617/chapter/1.

17 "Sleep Drive and Your Body Clock," Sleep Foundation, accessed September 15, 2015, https://sleepfoundation.org/sleep-topics/sleep-drive-and-your-body-clock.

wake up. When it's dark, your body releases melatonin, which helps ease it into sleep.

Why is sleep important? Here are a few reasons:

1.  Sleep is a time for rest and repair. Melatonin is also a powerful antioxidant and does a lot of work scavenging for free radicals at night.[18]

2.  Adequate sleep helps to control our carbohydrate cravings. In *Lights Out,* authors Wiley and Formby explain that our bodies are constantly thinking that it is summer because of the advent of artificial light. So when we stay up late and watch Netflix into the wee hours, this can suppress leptin (commonly thought of as the satiety hormone), causing us to continue to want to eat carbohydrates.[19]

3.  Jeff Iliff, in his TED Talk *One More Reason to Get a Good Night's Sleep,* speaks of the brain creating metabolic waste every day. It's only through sleep where the cerebrospinal fluid can flow into the brain and drain out this waste.[20] Pretty important, I think!

4.  Sleep is vital for memory formation, not only in our minds as what we remember, but also in the body as what our immune system remembers on a cellular level.[21]

One of my vices is to stream TV late into the night. I have super-busy days and often get home late and tired, and I like to zone out in front of the computer. Thus, I'm often staying up much later than I intended and falling asleep with the lights on. I find it to be a bad habit. When I do have the mind-set of simply closing my computer and turning off the lights, I always feel more rested and happy the next day.

18 "Melatonin," accessed September 15, 2015, http://www.lifeextension.com.

19 Wiley, T. S., and Bent Formby. *Lights Out: Sleep, Sugar, and Survival.* New York: Pocket Books, 2000.

20 "One More Reason to Get a Good Night's Sleep," YouTube video, filmed Sept 2014, http://www.ted.com/talks/jeff_iliff_one_more_reason_to_get_a_good_night_s_sleep?language=en.

21 Rasch, Björn, and Jan Born. "About Sleep's Role in Memory." *Physiological Reviews.* April 1, 2013, http://www.ncbi.nlm.nih.gov/pubmed/23589831.

Here are some simple things that both my clients and I work on to promote better sleep.

**MAKE YOUR BEDROOM A DARK HAVEN.** One of the simplest things you can do is to get dark shades that shut out light! My clients report this as being extremely helpful. Especially for those of us that live in urban centers, light pollution is a problem. This also means covering any blinking lights you have, or better yet, unplug them!

**TAKE OUT THE ELECTRONICS!** Playing on your phone or watching videos late at night can be very stimulating, making it harder to go to sleep. In addition, Ann Louise Gittleman has a great book called *Zapped*, where she talks about all the possible consequences from all those electronics we use. Certain people are very sensitive, and they find when they remove electronics from their bedroom, they get better sleep! I personally put my cell phone on airplane mode and try to leave my computer in the living room.

**DAB ON SOME LAVENDER ESSENTIAL OIL OR BODY SPRAY.** In one study, lavender was shown to help increase sleep in both men and women.[22]

**BE MINDFUL OF YOUR CAFFEINE INTAKE THROUGHOUT THE DAY.** Caffeine has a half-life of roughly six hours, meaning that it takes six hours for caffeine to fall to one-half of its potency. It takes caffeine 12 hours to completely leave your system. Having a cup in the morning shouldn't be a problem, but later on in the afternoon it could affect your sleep.

**GET SOME EXERCISE.** Exercise has been shown to improve sleep!

**TAKE A LITTLE MAGNESIUM.** Magnesium is one of the few supplements with many studies to back up its effectiveness.[23]

22 Goel, Namni, Hyungsoo Kim, and Raymund P. Lao. "An Olfactory Stimulus Modifies Nighttime Sleep in Young Men and Women." *Chronobiology International* 22, no. 5 (2009): 889–904, doi:10.1080/07420520500263276.

23 Abbasi, Behnood, Masud Kimiagar, Khosro Sadeghniiat, Minoo M. Shirazi, Mehdi Hedayati, and Bahram Rashidkhani. "The Effect of Magnesium Supplementation on Primary Insomnia in Elderly: A Double-blind Placebo-controlled Clinical Trial." *Journal of Research Medical Sciences* 17, no. 12 (2012), http://www.ncbi.nlm.nih.gov/pmc/articles/PMC3703169/.

The Nourished Soul and Body

Taking 200 to 400 milligrams of magnesium citrate or glycinate before bed can help relax the nervous system and muscles.

Sleep, like everything else, is just a small part of the equation. If it's something that speaks to you to work on, try getting to sleep a little earlier tonight, and see how it goes!

## Environment

We live in a very polluted world, much of which you can't control, but what you can control is what you put on your skin and what you use to clean your house.

The skin is extremely absorbent, and one way to introduce toxins into the body is through your skin-care products. There are a lot of numbers out there on how many beauty products people use, but from what I can observe through friends and family, even those that are pretty minimalist use one or two on a daily basis.

Have you looked at the ingredients label of your shampoo or your lotion? The FDA doesn't regulate what goes into beauty products, so there is very little oversight over what we are actually using. A great resource is the Environmental Working Group's Skin Deep Database. They rate many products that you normally see in the grocery store, and they have a downloadable app that you can use when you are at the store.

I personally have started making my own dry shampoo from arrowroot powder, and only use coconut oil on my skin. I find that I love the smell, and it absorbs really well. A good rule of thumb is not to put anything on your skin that you wouldn't eat!

The Environmental Working Group (EWG) also has a database of house cleaners, and a common brand like Formula 409 gets an F rating! According to the EWG, the ingredient in Formula 409, ethanolamine, creates moderate concern for respiratory conditions! No thank you. An old but great method to clean your countertops is to use one part water to one part white vinegar. Put it in a spray bottle and you're done.

So think about true nourishment in terms of everything that surrounds you. From the lotions and creams you put on your skin to what you are spraying on your countertops, think about replacing one thing at a time and you'll be well on your way.

## Hydration

One very important crucial piece of the Nourished Belly Diet and probably one of the simplest pieces to put in place is to drink more water. Most people I've met do not drink enough of it. Data analyzed in 2013 from 3,397 adults surveyed in 2007 had this breakdown: 7 percent of adults reported no daily consumption of drinking water, 36 percent reported drinking 1 to 3 cups, 35 percent reported drinking 4 to 7 cups, and 22 percent reported drinking 8 cups or more.[24] Even though these numbers aren't the MOST recent, it's unlikely behavior has changed all that much. There's always room for improvement!

Let's talk about a few reasons why water is so important.

- Think of blood as a way that nutrients are carried throughout the body and think of water as a very large component of blood.[25] When you don't drink enough water, you aren't giving your circulatory system enough building blocks to deliver all the nutrients you need in an efficient way.

- The electrolytes in your body need the medium of water to make reactions happen.

- Water lubricates your joints! For me, this is particularly important because I'm an athlete, and I plan to move for the rest of my life. Nothing puts a damper on your ability to move more than joint pain. The synovial fluid that encapsulates your joints is made primarily of water, so the more hydrated you are, the more protection you give your joints.

24 Goodman, Alyson B., Heidi M. Blanck, Bettylou Sherry, Sohyun Park, Linda Nebeling, and Amy L. Yaroch. "Behaviors and Attitudes Associated With Low Drinking Water Intake Among US Adults, Food Attitudes and Behaviors Survey, 2007." *Preventing Chronic Disease* (2013), http://dx.doi.org/10.5888/pcd10.120248.

25 "Plasma," American Red Cross, accessed September 15, 2015, http://www.redcrossblood .org/learn-about-blood/blood-components/plasma.

- Water helps regulate your temperature. You sweat; most other animals do not. Most of us have seen dogs panting away, and it's something rather remarkable that you can continue to move and be active in hot temperatures because your body has this ability to sweat and regulate temperature.

There are more reasons why water is the boss, but suffice it to say that you need to drink more of it! Another bonus is that you can include herbal teas (refer to Appendix E on page 204 for a beginning guide to herbal teas), bone broth, and veggie broth in your hydration mission.

||||||||||||||||||||||||||||||||||||||||||||||||||||||||||||||||||||||||||||||||||||||||||||||||||||||||||||||||

**NOURISHING NOTE:** Drink half your weight in ounces, and add 8 ounces for every 30 minutes of physical activity.

||||||||||||||||||||||||||||||||||||||||||||||||||||||||||||||||||||||||||||||||||||||||||||||||||||||||||||||||

## Nourishing Foods

You are here to discover what I mean by nourishing food—the main purpose of this book! As you read on, you'll learn more about eating regenerative foods that make deposits, how to use belly boosters, and which foods are uniquely meant for you.

# Holistic Health Assessment

The Nourished Belly Diet, as you are beginning to see, is not just about what you put into your mouth. It's about the way you live your life and the frame of mind in which you live it.

It's time to take a quick quiz. I love taking quizzes! They are always so informative. Below you'll find an assessment that I often give to clients to just check what's going on. I find it helpful to look at this assessment frequently to be reminded about a habit I might have let go of unintentionally or to find inspiration on what to work on next. Have a look at where you are starting from and what things you might want to work on first.

| Health Questions | Often | Seldom | Never |
| --- | --- | --- | --- |
| Do you eat out? | | | |
| Do you cook at home? | | | |
| Do you drink 2 liters of water a day? | | | |
| Do you eat vegetables 3 to 5 times a day? | | | |
| Do you have an effortless bowel movement every day? | | | |
| Do you know what you are going to eat before you get hungry? | | | |
| Do you take less than half an hour for meals? | | | |
| Do you know where your food comes from? (Where it's grown or raised?) | | | |
| Do you watch TV or work while you eat? | | | |
| Do you think about chewing? | | | |
| Do you smoke? | | | |
| Do you get less than seven hours of sleep a night? | | | |
| Do you sit most of the day? | | | |
| Do you exercise? | | | |
| Do you eat foods that are in packages? | | | |
| Do you spend time doing a creative hobby or art form? | | | |
| Do you spend quality time with friends and family? | | | |
| Do you feel stressed? | | | |
| Do you treat yourself to massages or healing appointments? | | | |
| Do your actions differ from your intentions? | | | |

The Nourished Soul and Body  27

| Mind-set Questions | Often | Seldom | Never |
|---|---|---|---|
| Do you look forward to your day when you wake up? | | | |
| Do you use the word "can't"? | | | |
| Do you often wish things were different? | | | |
| Do you laugh? | | | |
| Do you feel like you sacrifice in your life? | | | |
| Do you take risks? | | | |

Regardless of what you answered on this questionnaire, this is feedback for you. These are by no means all of the questions that could be asked, nor are they judgments. If a question brings some feelings up, that's informative. No one else knows why this is so, except for you.

What are areas that are growing edges for you? Keep a list of areas that you'd like to work on.

Keep this information in your back pocket as you read through this book. When you come to the Weekly Action Planner (page 81), you'll have an opportunity to create an action step around one of these lifestyle habits.

# 3

# Bank Your Body

I love working with food because it's a necessity every single day. I recently participated in a fast, and whoa was that interesting. Previously, I was not a big fan of fasts, but now I see that they have their benefits. My nutrition school founder, Ed Bauman, was running the program and he said something beautiful about emptying—both emptying the mind and emptying the body. After experiencing a week with just vegetable broth and juices, I see now how that can be powerful. It was interesting just to watch my hunger levels and spurts of energy and simply take part in an exercise of the mind. I also realized that much of my munching habits were just that...they were habits. It was a good experience.

Although there are benefits to fasting, it also made me see how important food really is. The entire week was pretty much devoid of fat and had very little protein. I came back feeling very, very depleted. My sleep was not as deep by the end of the week; I was very foggy and forgetful, and my libido was zero! The day after I got back, I tried to choreograph a three-minute song, and I could only dance for three minutes! It took all my energy. I slowly resumed eating regularly, and it took me three to four days to begin feeling strong again.

Yay to eating food! Really. I feel grateful every day that I get to work with food and share it with others. Simply posting a picture on Instagram gives me joy.

I personally love to nerd out on *everything* about food, from the fact that what we choose to eat can be as much a political statement as a personal one, to helpful ways to transform our views about food. Read on if you are a food nerd!

# Deposits and Withdrawals

This is one of the most helpful ways I look at what I eat and how I teach my clients to look at food. Food can either be regenerative and be *deposits,* or degenerative and be *withdrawals.* Think of your body as bank account where you have an account that grows with every deposit of nutrient-rich food. On the opposite side, there are foods that make withdrawals. Refined foods and sugar deplete your body of vitamins and minerals. Just like an account, if you continually make withdrawals, we will eventually be at zero, and unfortunately, this bank doesn't give you overdraft protection. This sets up the perfect environment for disease.

Below is a simple chart of some sample foods that are considered deposits and sample foods that are considered withdrawals. Now, The Nourished Belly Diet is not entirely made up of deposit foods, and I do not think any diet should be, unless you are battling with disease.

You've probably heard of the 80/20 rule, which I think is so helpful to aim for. Translating this into meals, think about 17 out of 21 meals you eat a week being amazing and the other four, allow for indulgences. That way, you are still building up your bank account so that when you make a withdrawal once in a while, it's not so bad. You have a cushion!

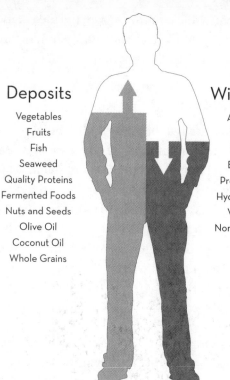

### Deposits

Vegetables
Fruits
Fish
Seaweed
Quality Proteins
Fermented Foods
Nuts and Seeds
Olive Oil
Coconut Oil
Whole Grains

### Withdrawals

Added Sugars
White Flour
Fried Foods
Baked Goods
Processed Foods
Hydrogenated Oils
Vegetable Oil
Non-Organic Foods
Candy

# Degenerative Foods

This section isn't to label foods as "bad" or pass judgments on anyone who happens to be eating cake as you read this book. The underlying reason to talk about withdrawal foods is to realize that they are degenerative. They may taste amazing, but if you indulge too much and they are too much a part of your diet, then you aren't truly nourishing yourself. With this knowledge and the initial goal of adding regenerative foods into the diet, you'll see that these foods will naturally start to slip way.

The withdrawal food that calls to me the most is a scone from Arizmendi, a local bakery that is steps away from where I live. I can get into the habit of taking a midday coffee and scone break. Also, plantain chips. Once I start eating them, it's really hard for me to not eat them every day.

So what's the big deal? Well, coming back to the idea of foods that make withdrawals, they don't give much nourishment, and when you eat them on a regular basis, lack of nutrition can be a stress on your body.

Let's take the scone, for example.

White flour and sugar are two of the main ingredients in scones. White flour, originally coming from the wholesome wheat berry, has been stripped of all its nutrients and is pure starch. Ann Louise Gittleman, in her book, *Get the Sugar Out*, writes that white flour is stripped of 22 vitamins and minerals in its processing.[26] Without fiber and nutrients, your body has to do very little to digest this scone, so it changes the flour to glucose rather quickly. Your blood sugar shoots up and as you'll read below, consistently high blood sugar is a bad thing.

## Sugar

Oh, sugar. More and more info is coming out about sugar and its effects, so I really try to moderate my sugar intake. It's a slippery slope, however, because I notice that as soon as I have some, I start to crave it regularly. Does that happen to you? When I was younger I was definitely addicted sugar. I used to steal things from the pantry and hide them in my room. As an adult not so long ago, I used to pour sugar in my coffee for five seconds. That's a *really* long time.

Today, I still struggle with sugar addiction and with the science coming out about sugar, it makes sense. Sugar triggers a dopamine release every single time you have it,[27] and it can activate the same pleasure pathways as opium and marijuana. So when you are feeling down, it makes you feel good! An entire book can be written about sugar (and there are many) and why it's important to clear

26  Gittleman, Ann Louise. *Get the Sugar Out: 501 Simple Ways to Cut the Sugar in Any Diet*. New York: Crown Trade Paperbacks, 1996.

27  Rada, P., N.M. Avena, and B.G. Hoebel. "Daily Bingeing on Sugar Repeatedly Releases Dopamine in the Accumbens Shell." *Neuroscience* 134, no. 3 (2005): 737-44, doi:10.1016/j. neuroscience.2005.04.043.

most of it from your life. I'm not going to get into everything here, but some important takeaway points are:

**IT CAN MAKE YOU FAT!** We tend to store many of the calories from sugar, instead of burning them. A great resource about sugar is Dr. Robert Lustig's book *Fat Chance*, which does an excellent job of explaining how we metabolize sugar in the body.

**IT CAN INTERFERE WITH MEMORY AND LEARNING.** Studies show that sugar lowers Brain Derived Neurotrophic Factor (BDNF). BDNF helps our brains create new neural connections to learn and remember new things.

**OVERUSE OF SUGAR CAN LEAD TO INSULIN RESISTANCE, WHICH CAN LEAD TO TYPE 2 DIABETES.** The more foods you eat that hit your bloodstream relatively quickly, the more your body has to work to keep your blood sugar stable. To do this, the pancreas releases insulin when it detects your blood sugar levels are too high. Insulin tells your body to sweep the sugar (glucose) into your cells for later use. This system can become overworked and can eventually lead to insulin resistance.

**SUGAR FEEDS UNHEALTHY BACTERIA AND YEASTS.** Your good bacteria love to eat certain things, and your bad bacteria does as well! When you eat a diet high in refined sugars, you feed only certain populations of bacteria and yeast, which don't particularly benefit our individual biomes.

## Trans Fats

There's debate now around which fats are good and which ones are bad, but pretty much everyone can agree that trans fats are no good. You'll find them in hydrogenated vegetable oils, which are solid at room temperature. The product that you are probably most familiar with is margarine. Yes, you remember, the alternative to butter that was touted as heart healthy? It turns out it's really not that good for you.

Margarine has an extremely interesting history—did you know it was originally gray? People generally found it unappealing, so they dyed it yellow to look like butter. Nina Planck, in her book *Real Food: What to Eat and Why*, provides the recipe for margarine, and it's pretty unappetizing. Plus, now we know it's a trans fat!

Margarine is not the only place that trans fats show up. If you happen to be looking at a packaged good, look for the words "partially hydrogenated" or "hydrogenated." Even though the label says "no trans fats," if the ingredients include these words, stay away! Food companies can say that a serving has zero trans fats when it has less than one-half gram. So, tiny loophole.

In general, I stay away from vegetable oils. A nutrition classmate of mine, Tess, once put it brilliantly. Don't use oil from food that is not normally oily. Take olives. They are pretty darn oily. Avocados too. Lots of oil! Animal fat. Super naturally oily! Coconuts? Crazy oily! But corn? Soy? Meh...not so much. Want more info? Don't worry, we'll talk more about fats later on.

# Alcohol

I was blessed by Asian genes: I get pretty itchy when I drink alcohol, and the Asian "glow" is guaranteed to happen. Plus, I get very sleepy almost immediately and a headache hits soon after. So alcohol has never really been my thing. I realize, however, that I am in the small minority of adults that do not drink. When I go into a bar, it always strikes me: "This is where all the adults hang out!"

How much alcohol is too much? Well, I realize that this is a very personal answer, partly because everyone has a different reaction to alcohol based on their genes, body weight, and habits. However, let's take a moment to look at what alcohol generally does to the body.

After you ingest alcohol, about 10 percent is absorbed in the stomach, 10 percent hits the brain (this is where those intoxicating effects set in), and the rest goes to the liver to finish metabolizing. In the liver, the alcohol is transformed into acetaldehyde, and then for those of you that have the enzyme acetaldehyde dehydrogenase (ALDH), which I and many other Asians do not possess, this acetaldehyde is converted into acetic acid radicals and expelled. Acetaldehyde, if not converted, is a toxic by-product and can cause liver damage.

Another interesting note is that majority of the calories from your alcohol are stored rather than used. In his book *Fat Chance,* Dr. Robert Lustig explains that the way we metabolize alcohol and fructose are very similar, where larger portions of calories are metabolized through the liver and stored as fat for later. This fat is often stored as subcutaneous fat (under the skin) and surrounds organs, where it may not be visible but is thought to increase the likelihood of disease.

The last point I'll cover is that oftentimes, people have a drink to relax and get to bed, but studies actually show our sleep is less restful on alcohol.[28]

# Regenerative Foods

Now for the fun part! You are at the point in the book when I actually talk about what foods are great to eat! This next section is on regenerative foods, the backbone of the Nourished Belly Diet. I'll explain why they are so powerful and delicious at the same time.

The number one thing that you are trying to do with the Nourished Belly Diet is come back to whole foods. A whole food is anything that isn't processed in a large factory before it arrives on your plate. No need to read labels or throw away packaging; just eat it raw, sauté, bake, boil, or put it in the slow cooker. Done.

Take a stroll around the outskirts of the grocery store for the freshest produce or walk through a farmers market, or even shop from online retailers that source directly from farmers to expand your world of whole foods. There are plenty of new fruits and vegetables out there waiting to be discovered and

28 "Alcohol and Sleep—Alcohol Alert No. 41-1998." National Institute on Alcohol Abuse and Alcoholism. Last modified July 1, 1998. Accessed September 16, 2015, http://pubs.niaaa.nih.gov/publications/aa41.htm.

eaten! Biologically, we want variety so that we can have all of the nutrients that we need.

## SOUL Foods:
## Seasonal, Organic, Unrefined, and Local

At the very least, I do my best to follow the SOUL guidelines. Regenerative foods are Seasonal, Organic, Unrefined, and Local. Sometimes following these isn't always possible, but to the best of my ability I adhere to these ideas:

SEASONAL: When you find a tomato, or an apple in February, more often than not these are shipped long distances to get to you. By eating foods that are in season, you'll get more nutrients and you'll save on greenhouse gases too. Are you unsure of how to buy in season? Below you'll find a rough guide. Of course, what foods are available depend largely on which part of the world/country you live in; the information below is based on US growing seasons. This is by no means exhaustive, but this will give you a general idea.

| US Growing Seasons | | | |
|---|---|---|---|
| Spring | Summer | Fall | Winter |
| Asparagus | Peaches | Winter squash | Kale |
| Beets | Pears | Citrus | Collard greens |
| Onions | Tomatoes | Broccoli | Potatoes |
| Peas | Cucumbers | Cauliflower | Brussels sprouts |
| Strawberries | Watermelons | Apples | Cabbage |
| Berries | Peppers | Pears | Carrots |
| Nettles | Eggplant | Persimmons | Kohlrabi |
| Cherries | Beans | | |
| | Summer squash | | |
| | Melons | | |
| | Corn | | |
| | Eggs (Yes, eggs are seasonal!) | | |
| | Artichokes | | |
| | Figs | | |
| | Garlic | | |

*The* Nourished Belly Diet

The best way to buy in season is to buy directly from farmers. I love how it makes eating so much more enjoyable. I get super excited when it's peach or blackberry season, and when winter squashes come out, and then cherries and tomatoes—the list goes on and on. I'm sure you've seen fruits that aren't in season at the grocery store, and they are mad expensive! When you buy in season, you also buy what's plentiful, and therefore reasonably priced.

ORGANIC: I often get asked what the difference is between organic and conventional foods. A lot of people think that organic just means a higher price tag, and it's true, organic foods are a bit pricier, and sometimes a lot pricier. I find that the benefits I get from buying things organic, not only based on taste, is that I can ensure good practices at the level of production—for the most part. It tends to get a bit complicated as we see large-scale organic companies, but in general, it's a good thing.

A great resource to understand how most of the farmland in this country is used is *The Omnivore's Dilemma* by Michael Pollan. To sum it up very briefly, the vast majority of conventional farms rotate between very few crops and use chemical fertilizer and spray with pesticides (you've probably heard of Roundup and the genetically modified seeds that are "Roundup ready.") There are policies in the US government that support this way of farming, with subsidies on certain crops.

Organic, for the most part, provides a better alternative. Here's a few assurances you receive when you buy organic:

1. Land management practices maximize the health of soil and of the groundwater.

2. No pesticides or fertilizers are used that have synthetic chemicals.

3. All seeds must be organic (there are some exceptions here), but this also means that seeds cannot be genetically modified. (See page 39 for more info on GMOs.)

4. Animals are provided with living conditions that "accommodate health and natural behavior of animals... continuous total confinement of animals indoors is prohibited."[29]

5. Animals are fed organic feed where no antibiotics are routinely added.

6. No hormones are allowed to promote growth.

It's actually a crazy exercise to read through some of the organic standards, because they also have stipulations like, "no plastic pellets will be used in feed for roughage," and "no poultry slaughter by-products will be fed to poultry." Which means, that if it's written into the law, then people had been using those practices in conventional farming! Yuck!

The complete list of standards can be found on the USDA website.

‖‖‖‖‖‖‖‖‖‖‖‖‖‖‖‖‖‖‖‖‖‖‖‖‖‖‖‖‖‖‖‖‖‖‖‖‖‖‖‖‖‖‖‖‖‖‖‖‖‖‖‖‖‖‖‖‖‖‖‖‖‖‖‖‖‖‖‖‖‖‖‖‖‖‖‖‖‖‖‖‖‖‖‖‖

**NOURISHING NOTE:** Be wary of words on packaged boxes.

- Terms like "free range," "cage free," or "natural" don't have any real meaning and have no third-party certifiers. Companies are free to use these words as they choose, so be discerning!

- I don't buy organic from China or Mexico. There is much less oversight in these countries—so it's not as reliable what you are going to get. However, according to the CCOF (California Certified Organic Farmers) website, Mexico just finalized organic standards and CCOF-certified sites will need to comply by April 2015.[30] So that's a good sign.

‖‖‖‖‖‖‖‖‖‖‖‖‖‖‖‖‖‖‖‖‖‖‖‖‖‖‖‖‖‖‖‖‖‖‖‖‖‖‖‖‖‖‖‖‖‖‖‖‖‖‖‖‖‖‖‖‖‖‖‖‖‖‖‖‖‖‖‖‖‖‖‖‖‖‖‖‖‖‖‖‖‖‖‖‖

---

29 "Part 205: National Organic Program." ECFR – Code of Federal Regulations. September 15, 2015. Accessed September 16, 2015, http://www.ecfr.gov/cgi-bin/retrieveECFR?gp=1&SID=3001f6d7ca4a354fd78532eb75f5ebcf&ty=HTML&h=L&mc=true&n=pt7.3.205&r=PART.

30 "Mexico Organic Standards Finalized." CCOF Inc., January 8, 2014, accessed September 16, 2015, http://www.ccof.org/mexico-organic-standards-finalized.

# What's the big deal with GMOs?

Apparently, the USDA's definition of GMOs is actually different than what most of the rest of the world thinks.

Definition of a GMO from the World Health Organization website:

Genetically modified organisms (GMOs) can be defined as organisms (i.e., plants, animals, or microorganisms) in which the genetic material (DNA) has been altered in a way that does not occur naturally by mating and/or natural recombination. The technology is often called "modern biotechnology" or "gene technology," sometimes also "recombinant DNA technology" or "genetic engineering." It allows selected individual genes to be transferred from one organism into another, also between nonrelated species. Foods produced from or using GM organisms are often referred to as GM foods.

The USDA's definition of genetic engineering is: Manipulation of an organism's genes by introducing, eliminating, or rearranging specific genes using the methods of modern molecular biology, particularly those techniques referred to as recombinant DNA techniques.[31]

The USDA's definition of GMOs is: The production of heritable improvements in plants or animals for specific uses, via either genetic engineering or other more traditional methods.

I prefer the WHO's definition, where it simply refers to genetic engineering. The USDA definition could include selective breeding of crops, which in my mind, is vastly different from inserting DNA of unrelated species into the gene sequencing of plants.

Since we are in the US, I will use the term genetic engineering instead of GMO to be clear. Is genetic engineering good for us? Currently, there is just not enough research out there to say definitively yes or no. However, here are my two cents:

---

[31] "Glossary of Agricultural Biotechnology Terms," Biotechnology Glossary, February 27, 2013, accessed September 16, 2015, http://www.usda.gov/wps/portal/usda/usdahome?navid=BIOTECH_GLOSS&navtype=RT&parentnav=BIOTECH.

There haven't been any long-term studies on the long-term effects of eating genetically engineered food. However, one of the more common talking points that you'll hear has to do with seeds that are resistant to the herbicide Roundup. They are genetically engineered to withstand being sprayed with this chemical, whose job is to kill weeds around it. A major component of Roundup is a chemical called glyphosate. In March 2015, the cancer research branch of the World Health Organization, the IARC (Internation Agency for Research on Cancer), labeled glyphosate as *probably carcinogenic to humans*.[32] Plus, California's EPA intends to include glyphosate on its list of chemicals known to cause cancer. There is of course debate from the makers and users of glyphosate, but if I had to choose, I would choose foods without the chemicals that probably cause cancer.

With everything I have control over, I strive to choose the cleanest food possible. If I had the choice, I would prefer that my food not be genetically engineered.

**UNREFINED:** This is a call to eat whole foods and stay away from processed, packaged foods. In terms of health and weight loss, those of my clients that move away from eating anything that has a label invariably feel a whole lot better. We all fall prey at times to eating foods because we need something convenient and quick, but the more we can become accustomed to packing a whole foods snack, and making sure our meals are from whole foods, the better we'll feel.

**LOCAL:** When we buy locally produced food, we support our own local economy and don't pay the transportation costs associated with foods that are shipped in from far away. Plus, we automatically buy foods that are in season when we buy local produce. I also like to buy from local companies for the same reasons. These items

---

32 "IARC Monographs Volume 112: Evaluation of Five Organophosphate Insecticides and Herbicides," International Agency for Research on Cancer, March 20, 2015, http://www.iarc.fr/en/media-centre/iarcnews/pdf/MonographVolume112.pdf.

tend to be fresher and use fewer preservatives than a product that needs to sit on a grocery shelf.

Remember, again, that our dollars have power, and where we spend our money is powerful. According to the American Independent Business Alliance, there is something called the multiplier effect, where when you spend a dollar at a local business, more of that dollar will stay in the community as opposed to when you spend it at a franchise.[33]

If I can, I buy at farmers markets or small grocery stores. I do shop at Whole Foods from time to time, more for nonperishables (canned fish, for example), but I find that local grocery stores have pretty good deals on produce. Farmers markets, for me, are an enjoyable way to spend an afternoon, and I prefer to support farmers directly. A lot of farmers use sustainable practices, but aren't certified organic. The certification process can be expensive, which can be a barrier for some farmers to certify themselves. So, you should ask the farmer if they use pesticides or commercial fertilizers.

I make exceptions for coconut oil/milk, ginger, sea salt, spices, and chocolate! Many of these things cannot be grown close to me, and historically, we've traded for staples. However, when I make exceptions, I look for terms like fair trade, non-GMO, and organic. You can find out more about these labels in the Recommended Resources (page 208).

## Bone Broth

What makes *The Nourished Belly Diet* slightly different from other diet books is that at its foundation are traditional foods such as bone broth. Broth, an extremely mineral-rich food found in culinary traditions around the world, is at the base of many recipes of *The Nourished Belly Diet*. It's one of the first must-have foods that I introduce to clients when they are looking to make

---

33 "The Multiplier Effect of Local Independent Businesses," AMIBA, April 15, 2015, accessed September 16, 2015, http://www.amiba.net/resources/multiplier-effect/.

a big change in what they eat. Thank goodness, too, because it actually makes eating extremely delicious.

Bone broth is as traditional as it gets. You'll find a bone broth–based soup or stew in pretty much any culture's culinary cuisine. It's often prescribed to build up strength, and it's at the foundation of the popular GAPS (Gut and Psychology Syndrome) diet for those who need to rebuild their gut lining. Let's take a look at why it's so powerful.

**HIGH IN MINERALS.** Due to the lack of minerals in soils on conventional farms and the current American state of health, most people are deficient in minerals. Minerals are just as important as vitamins to our daily bodily functions. Bones are a powerhouse of minerals. In *Nourishing Broth,* Kaayla Daniel and Sally Fallon Morell state that bones are made up of 50 percent mineral content.[34] Through prolonged simmering, you can extract all of these precious nutrients. Thomas Cowan, author of *The Fourfold Path to Healing,* suggests that adding bone broth to your diet is the fastest way to rebuild your mineral deposits.

**AN IMPORTANT SOURCE OF GELATIN.** Bone broth does not always come out gelatinous, since it depends on the age of the animal and the way you make your broth. But when your broth gels when cooled, you know you have liquid gold! Gelatin is the culinary word for collagen, and collagen is what makes up 25 to 35 percent of the body's total protein.[35] Collagen is responsible for holding your body together—literally. It acts as the glue that holds your muscles, joints, and cell structures in place. You can think of the glue as losing its effectiveness as you age, and thus you can break apart more easily. Not an awesome image, but makes sense, right?

While I was researching bone broth and learning its benefit to joint health, the athlete in me immediately took bones out of the freezer and started making a batch. You don't realize what a

---

34 Fallon, Sally, and Kaayla T. Daniel. *Nourishing Broth: An Old-fashioned Remedy for the Modern World.* New York: Grand Central Lifestyle, 2014.

35 Ibid.

blessing joint health is until one fails you. Your joints give you the option to bend, squat, and walk—essential motions for everyday life. One of the primary ways your joints are protected is with the synovial fluid that surrounds your joint cavities. Through movement, synovial fluid moves in and out of the joint capsule while providing nutrients you need to maintain joint health and also cushioning your joints from impact.

Hydration and optimum nutrition are important to this process. One way to maintain all the different components of synovial fluid is to drink plenty of broth. Broth, especially gelatinous broth, is full of the building blocks of synovial fluid. You've probably heard of the effectiveness of glucosamine and chondroitin sulfate when it comes to joint health. Broth provides natural sources of both of these nutrients.

**HEALING AND REGENERATIVE.** Gelatinous broth is an excellent digestive aid and is extremely healing to your gut, nervous system, and entire body. This is the original reason that Jell-O is served in hospitals. Patients were served a gelatin-based food, but in the words of *Full Moon Feast* author Jessica Prentice, the Jell-O served to patients nowadays to patients is a "toxic mimic" of tradition.

Broth is not a complete protein, primarily missing tryptophan, but it has some important amino acids. Included in the large amino acid profile of bone broth are glycine, proline, and glutamine.

- **GLYCINE** is necessary in creating glucose when you are in need of more energy and is vital in supporting your detoxification pathways (thus, cleansing with only bone broth is a great idea).

- **PROLINE** is essential for the production of collagen, which helps maintain healthy skin, bones, ligaments, tendons, and cartilage.

- **GLUTAMINE** is important for gut health, as it helps to feed enterocytes, which absorb digested food and transport nutrients to the bloodstream. Glutamine helps to keep the integrity of the gut lining, which is now seen as preventing food allergies and possibly being tied to mood disorders.

Bone broth can be used by itself as a snack, with a little miso, and is a fabulous base for soups and stews. I suggest my clients use it instead of water to cook rice or any grain. Adding just a splash to stir-fries not only supplies nutrients, but flavor.

## Healthy Fat

Newsflash: Fat and cholesterol are no longer the enemies in our diets! This is great and incredible news, since fat is what carries the flavor in dishes, makes you feel satiated, and is necessary for you to absorb fat-soluble vitamins. Eating fat doesn't make you fat.

In regards to cholesterol, the 2015 *Dietary Guidelines for Americans* says that we shouldn't be concerned with dietary cholesterol:

> Previously, the *Dietary Guidelines for Americans* recommended that cholesterol intake be limited to no more than 300 mg/day. The 2015 *DGAC* will not bring forward this recommendation because available evidence shows no appreciable relationship between consumption of dietary cholesterol and serum cholesterol, consistent with the conclusions of the AHA/ACC report. Cholesterol is not a nutrient of concern for overconsumption.[36]

What!? This is huge! The American Heart Association (AHA) has said that the dietary amount of cholesterol in food has very little to do with changing how much cholesterol is in our blood. This means that we don't need to eat egg white omelettes anymore! Thank goodness! They really don't taste that great, am I right? Eating the whole egg, using coconut oil, and putting butter on your potatoes is back in! As someone who wants to *enjoy* their food, I consider fat a necessity for taste and satiety.

Now, there is still a lot of debate out there about the right kinds of fats, and which fats are good and which fats are bad. You'll find

---

36 "Scientific Report of 2015 Dietary Guidelines Committee,"[USDA], accessed September 16, 2015, http://health.gov/dietaryguidelines/2015-scientific-report/pdfs/scientific-report-of-the-2015-dietary-guidelines-advisory-committee.pdf.

all sorts of studies out there that support one camp or the other. I think what is safe to say is that you no longer have to avoid things like the plague. Eat a steak once in a while, but also eat plenty of fish, chicken, pork, coconut oil, walnuts, etc. If you have a healthy rotation happening, then you can be sure that you are varying the types of fats that you consume. Please refer to Appendix A to learn about which cooking oils are part of the Nourished Belly Diet!

Harold McGee, in one of my bibles, *On Food and Cooking*, says fat is essential because of its relationship with water. They do *not* mix, so in our bodies, fats form barriers that keep what we want in and what we don't want out. Cell membranes, for example, with the perfect mix of saturated fats, unsaturated fats, and cholesterol, allow nutrients to come in and out.

However, both from a culinary and nutritional perspective, fat is essential! Here's why:

- Carries the flavor. Many aromatic and flavor compounds are hydrophobic, meaning they are repelled by water. However, they love fat. Flavors are fat soluble and are carried throughout the dish in the fat molecules.

- Keeps foods moist. Ever had a super-dry piece of chicken?

- Crisping. Fat also gives that crispy brownness to food. One of my favorite things to do with leftover chicken skin is to put it in the pan and let it crisp up. Then I crumble it and put it over my stir-fry veggies. Yum!

- Provides a concentrated source of energy. After carbohydrates, our bodies will break down fats for energy. A gram of fat provides nine calories of energy as compared to four calories per gram of carbohydrate.

- Protects our organs and cells.

- Triggers satiation. Have you ever eaten a whole bag of crackers, or a whole bag of popcorn and felt like you didn't eat anything at all?

- Regulates body temperature.

- Carries important fat-soluble nutrients (Vitamins A, D, E, and K; carotenes; chlorophyll) in the body.

- Slows the digestion of carbohydrates into the blood.

- Provides the building blocks of hormones in the body.

## What's the deal with the omegas?

You've probably heard the word "omega-3s" thrown around a lot, and that certain foods have them, and they are good thing. What exactly are they?

There are lots of nutrients we can make ourselves. When foods are called "essential," it means that we cannot synthesize them in our own bodies. Two of the fatty acids that we cannot synthesize, which you've probably heard of, are omega-3s and omega-6s. These two different types of fatty acids are crucial to our bodies in many ways.

Essential fatty acids (EFAs) help maintain cell membrane fluidity and stability, and work in the development and function of brain and nerve tissue, oxygen transfer, energy production, immune functions, and conversion of compounds involved in all body functions.

Importantly, EFAs can either decrease or increase inflammation in the body. They are converted within the body into prostaglandins, which are hormone-like substances that help regulate the inflammatory response.

Omega-6s can lead to two types of prostaglandins, one that is inflammatory and one that is anti-inflammatory, while omega-3s lead to only anti-inflammatory substances in the body. Remember that your body needs both inflammation and the counter to have a healthy immune system and physiological responses. The following flow chart shows how acids we ingest from foods are converted into either omega-3s or omega-6s.

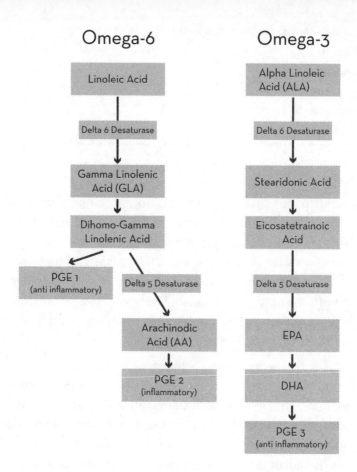

## Omega-6

Linoleic Acid

↓ Delta 6 Desaturase

Gamma Linolenic Acid (GLA)

↓

Dihomo-Gamma Linolenic Acid

→ PGE 1 (anti inflammatory)

Delta 5 Desaturase →

Arachinodic Acid (AA)

↓

PGE 2 (inflammatory)

## Omega-3

Alpha Linoleic Acid (ALA)

↓ Delta 6 Desaturase

Stearidonic Acid

↓

Eicosatetrainoic Acid

↓ Delta 5 Desaturase

EPA

↓

DHA

↓

PGE 3 (anti inflammatory)

In each of these pathways, there are steps where both omega-3s and omega-6s use the exact same enzymes, or catalysts that make things happen in the body. Therefore, they are competing for enzymes and must be eaten in the correct ratio. The Standard American Diet (SAD) currently has an extreme ratio of omega-6 to omega-3, and some sources even cite 40:1! The healthy range is anywhere from 4:1 or even 1:1.

So, if you are like most people, it's a pretty safe bet that you need to increase the amount of omega-3 in your diet. Here are some foods to focus on:

- Cold water fish (salmon, sardines)
- Flaxseed and flaxseed oil
- Chia seeds
- Pasture-raised beef and chicken
- Seafood
- Hemp seeds

## Veggies

According to the CDC, in 2011, California, Oregon, and New Hampshire had the highest amount of daily consumption of vegetables in all of the US, with the average being greater or equal to 1.8 servings a day.[37] Unfortunately, if that is what's topping the charts, we could do a lot better. There are, of course, issues of access both in supply and availability, but even when resources aren't the problem, most people aren't eating enough of the colorful stuff.

Once you start incorporating a lot of vegetables into your diet, it's hard to go back, because you start *feeling* really good. When I eat a lot of veggies, my energy is better, my bowel movements are fantastic, and I have a sense of lightness that I don't have when I'm eating out and eating a lot of processed foods. My clients that make the switch often comment that they start craving vegetables! This makes total sense because once you start giving the body what it needs, it will love you for it and start to ask for it.

In the Nourished Belly Diet, the focus is on dark, leafy greens and eating the rainbow. Part of this journey is to experiment, to eat veggies that you've never eaten before. I now love to eat all different types of kale, love when I see fresh nettles, and relish all of those Asian greens that I grew up on. I love making jicama salads and playing around with burdock, and have just discovered that I love kohlrabi! There are so many foods out there, and I find it joyful to eat something and say—what is this? It's amazing!

37 "State Indicator Report on Fruits and Vegetables 2013," National Center for Chronic Disease Prevention and Health Promotion, accessed September 16, 2015, http://www.cdc.gov/nutrition/downloads/State-Indicator-Report-Fruits-Vegetables-2013.pdf.

Vegetables are not only a source of fiber, vitamins, and minerals, but also antioxidants. Antioxidants are vital in regeneration because they stop oxidation from occurring in the body. Think of it like this: Regular bodily processes will create oxidation, or free radicals. Eating the wrong things, breathing in pollution, smoking, or being stressed will also create more oxidation or free radicals in the body. A free radical is a cell that is missing one electron, and therefore highly unstable. It will steal an electron from a healthy molecule, creating cell damage and more free radicals. The cycle goes on. Antioxidants are great because they just happen to have extra electrons and they love giving electrons away and healing the free radicals.

Colors are the sign that foods are full of antioxidants. For a complete guide to antioxidants, flip to Appendix B (page 191).

## Fermented Foods

Gut bacteria, gut flora, your microbiome—you'll hear these words if you are tapped into any health scene, and you are certain to hear more in the coming years. More and more information is coming out around the benefits of varied populations of bacteria. And thank goodness, because they are *everywhere,* from the skin, mouth, and digestive tract to the nether regions.

It turns out that you have more bacteria on your body than you do cells; bacteria outnumber cells 10:1. Your intestines alone have over 100 trillion bacteria. The sheer number is mind-boggling, but the variety of species is also amazing. In the mouth, there are estimates of thousands of separate species in saliva and plaque.[38]

The vagina is another place with a varied bacterial presence that protects the reproductive tract from potential pathogens. The main species that dominates the vagina is lactobacilli, which are thought to crowd out more pathogenic species. This is an important conversation to have, since it's estimated that one-third

---

38 Robinson, C. J., B. J. M. Bohannan, and V. B. Young. "From Structure to Function: The Ecology of Host-Associated Microbial Communities." *Microbiology and Molecular Biology Reviews* 74, no. 3 (2010): 453-76. Accessed September 16, 2015, doi:10.1128/MMBR.00014-10.

of women will experience bacterial vaginosis, where the balance of good and bad bacteria in the vagina is disrupted.

The bacteria in your intestines play an incredibly important role in digestion and nourishing your body. Remember those 100 trillion bacteria that reside in your guts? It seems that all these little guys do a *lot* for your health. We are still in early stages of studying everything they do, but research is coming out about the role they play with breaking down hard-to-digest nutrients, setting your metabolism, synthesizing B and K vitamins, producing neurotransmitters, and providing a protective barrier against invading pathogens.

The balance of good and bad bacteria help keep disease at bay. It helps to consume less of the foods, like sugar, that feed the harmful bacteria, take a good-quality probiotic, and start eating more fermented foods. Yum!

Many traditional cultures have fermented foods, and they are making a comeback and being reintroduced into the American palate. Wine, yogurt, and fermented meats were all a part of traditional diets. Fermented foods contain live bacteria that when eaten help add to the diversity of your own microbiome. Fermentation occurs when foods are placed in an anaerobic environment, or an environment without oxygen. You can do this at home by submerging what you'd like to ferment under water, and usually, adding sea salt to create an environment suitable for lactic acid bacteria.

The sourness of many ferments completes a dish, giving it a more rounded flavor, and adding a bit of sauerkraut or yogurt can help add to the complexity of a dish. The benefits of fermented foods include:

- Fermentation helps to preserve foods and makes certain nutrients more available. Fermenting grains, for example, helps to neutralize the nutrient-binding phytates. Soy and cacao are other examples of foods that need to be fermented before consumption.

- Fermented foods are *living* foods. Making them yourself ensures that you keep cultures alive. Watch out for commercially made ferments that are pasteurized, which kills any living bacteria.

- Beneficial bacteria keep bad bacteria and yeasts in check. You are in a constant battle with renegade bacteria and yeasts. Without your beneficial bacteria, these other opportunistic creatures attempt to take over. Antibiotic use is indiscriminate and wipes out *all* bacteria; eating fermented foods can aid in repopulating beneficial colonies.

## Ferments that you can make at home or buy

KOMBUCHA: Kombucha is a fermented drink that was the first soda; fermentation of tea and sugar creates a fizzy drink that is filled with probiotics. It's great for detoxing and adding in a healthy dose of beneficial bacteria. Making kombucha at home is simple and inexpensive. You can easily ask around to find a starter SCOBY (which stands for symbiotic community of bacteria and yeast), or buy one online. Kombucha might not be the best choice for people who are trying to avoid sugar, however, since the amount of sugar can vary depending on the length of time spent in fermentation.

YOGURT: People who are extremely sensitive to dairy can find yogurt bothersome, but others who are lactose intolerant can do fine since fermentation eats much of the lactose. The longer the yogurt ferments, the more lactose is eaten by bacteria and the tangier the yogurt. Making your own yogurt is extremely easy (Homemade Yogurt, page 101) and the best way to ensure a long ferment. Store-bought yogurts tend not to have the tanginess that I like. Be especially wary of buying flavored varieties, since many of them are extremely high in added sugar. Best to buy whole plain organic yogurt and add your own sweetener or mix with fresh or dried fruit.

MISO: Miso is made of fermented soybeans and full of that umami flavor. Umami is often thought of as the fifth flavor that contributes to mouthfeel and a savory taste. It's full of nutrients and makes a wonderful soup base. Be sure to buy organic, as most conventional soybeans are genetically modified. Miso makes a wonderful marinade, and one way to ensure that bacteria is alive is to use it cold in a salad dressing.

**SAUERKRAUT:** Sauerkraut is another very easy thing to make at home, but feel free to buy kraut at the store, preferably in a glass container (the acids in fermented foods can leach unpleasant chemicals from the plastic into your food). Check out how to make sauerkraut at home on page 98.

**TEMPEH:** Tempeh is another fermented soy product and is a great protein source for vegans and vegetarians. The fermenting makes the nutrients in soy more bioavailable (meaning that we absorb them very easily); plus, tempeh is great at taking on the flavor of any dish.

**KIMCHI:** This spicy fermented cabbage dish from Korea is a great addition to rice dishes and is another great way to add healthy bacteria into the diet.

**KEFIR:** Kefir is another fermented beverage; most varieties that you'll see in the grocery store will be dairy ferments, but you can add kefir grains to coconut milk, cow's milk, or juice. The kefir grains are slightly different for each, but it's another super-easy drink to add into the mix. It's easy to go online and find kefir starters.

## Belly Boosters

Belly boosters play an important supporting role. My nutrition school, Bauman College, calls them booster foods, and their philosophy about them is great. They can be added to any snack or meal for flavor and nutrients. When I work with clients, we slowly increase the amount of belly boosters that we keep in our kitchens so that eventually, we get to a place where we are always thinking of which belly booster to add for some crunch, some flavor, and an extra nutritional punch. These include seaweeds, nuts, herbs, and spices. For a detailed list of belly boosters, go to Appendix C.

## Individual Nourishing

One of the most important tenets of the Nourished Belly Diet is that what regenerates you could be horrible for someone else! We are all different. We all have different ancestry and different genes and grew up eating different things while surrounded by different environments. I would be doing a disservice if I said that one thing is the miracle food for anyone.

All this is to say that there *is* one diet that will work really well for you! When I work with clients, I take the time to find out foods that make them FEEL REALLY GOOD. Some clients take food sensitivity tests, but a lot of them figure it out through food journaling and just staying aware of how they feel after they eat. Many times people feel sleepy after a meal, or just run down, and they attribute it to not getting enough sleep the night before. Many even think that this feeling is normal after eating. A popular television show called *The Boondocks* called it the "itis," or we often say "food coma." This is not normal!

If you are serious about going on the journey of nourishing yourself through regenerative foods, take the time to figure out which foods work for you and which foods don't. How do you know if a food doesn't work for you? Well, look for bloating, gas, feeling tired, skin breakouts and rashes, and brain fog. If you have an idea that something bothers you, take it out for a week and see how you feel. Then add it back intentionally and monitor yourself for any symptoms. The most common foods that can cause people trouble are gluten, dairy, eggs, shellfish, peanuts, citrus, nuts, corn, and soy.

If you need help, you can always find a holistic health practitioner that can do some food sensitivity testing and give you a plan to follow an elimination diet.

# The Nourished Bowl

Sometimes it's helpful to have a visual representation of what a nourishing meal should look like. Pictured below is the Nourished Bowl. Not every meal will look like this, but it's a great target to shoot for. I tell my clients to eat out of bowls instead of plates because it's a lot easier to watch portion size. Search for the perfect bowl to meet your perfect meal size. The Nourished Bowl graphic is how I teach my clients to start thinking about their meals and even snacks. If you use the graphic as a general guide, you'll be doing a pretty good job of making sure you are getting all the nutrients you need.

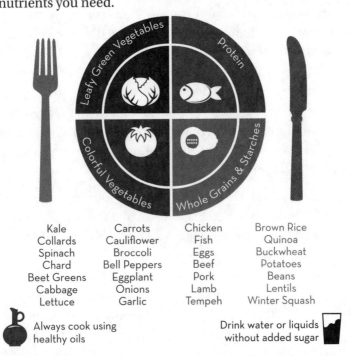

| | | | |
|---|---|---|---|
| Kale | Carrots | Chicken | Brown Rice |
| Collards | Cauliflower | Fish | Quinoa |
| Spinach | Broccoli | Eggs | Buckwheat |
| Chard | Bell Peppers | Beef | Potatoes |
| Beet Greens | Eggplant | Pork | Beans |
| Cabbage | Onions | Lamb | Lentils |
| Lettuce | Garlic | Tempeh | Winter Squash |

Always cook using healthy oils

Drink water or liquids without added sugar

Let's look at each piece of the Nourished Bowl carefully:

## Leafy Greens

Usually when I start working with clients, this is one of the main sections that are non-existent. When I say leafy greens, I mean the dark, thick ones, like kale, collards, spinach, beet greens, and mustard greens. Anything dark and leafy you can eat raw, but sautéing is also a great option. Remember that certain nutrients are enhanced with cooking, and some are destroyed, so eating a mix of cooked and raw is great! I tend to cook thicker leaves like kale and collards because I find I digest them better cooked.

When I look at the diet journals of clients, on average, vegetables come in the form of salads. I have nothing against salads, and in the summer, it seems that they are all I want to eat. Plus you can put a *lot* of things into a salad; but my point here is that putting a cup of lettuce on your plate doesn't really give you everything that you need. If I had the choice of eating a cup of cooked leafy greens over salad, I'd pretty much choose the dark greens every time.

Let's compare the nutrients from 100 grams of raw kale to 100 grams of lettuce. (Numbers from *The Encyclopedia of Healing Foods* by Michael Murray.)

|  | Kale | Lettuce |
|---|---|---|
| **Calories** | 50 | 18 |
| **Fiber** | 2 g | 1.9 g |
| **Calcium** | 135 mg | 68 mg |
| **Iron** | 1.7 mg | 1.4 mg |
| **Magnesium** | 34 mg | 11 mg |
| **Potassium** | 447 mg | 264 mg |
| **Vitamin A** | 8900 IU | 1900 IU |
| **Vitamin C** | 120 mg | 18 mg |
| **Vitamin K** | 817 mcg | 210 mcg |

Across the board, every nutrient is more substantial in kale than in lettuce. Yes, I would venture to say that the average American is feeling pretty good about their lettuce, and that's great! It's a first step. The next step is to explore the world of dark, leafy greens. The thicker, the better. Next time you go to the store, fondle some kale and compare it to lettuce. There's a big difference! Lettuce is great too, especially all the different kinds, but you want variety! The Nourished Bowl suggests a quarter of the bowl is filled with dark, leafy greens. Maybe that's something you are ready to take on?

||||||||||||||||||||||||||||||||||||||||||||||||||||||||||||||||||||||||||||||||||||||||||||||||

NOURISHING NOTE: Most dark, green leafy greens like spinach, chard, and beet greens have a very high amount of oxalates. Oxalates can be problematic for certain conditions and also tend to bind to minerals such as calcium and zinc,[39] making them unavailable for us. They are essentially sharp crystals that can build up in the kidneys and lead to kidney stones, but they can also build up in muscle tissue and make movement very painful. A dear friend of mine who has Lyme disease is very sensitive to oxalates. She reports feeling achy immediately after eating something high in them. Again, you don't need to avoid them completely unless you having something chronic happening, in which case experimenting with removing them could be a good idea. Variety is key!

||||||||||||||||||||||||||||||||||||||||||||||||||||||||||||||||||||||||||||||||||||||||||||||||

## Colorful Veggies

This is where vegetables of every other color go. Think carrots, tomatoes, eggplants, bell peppers—think the rainbow! These will also change with the seasons (refer to the seasonal chart on page 36) as will your dark greens, depending on where you live. Basically, whenever I make anything, I like to make sure that it's as colorful as possible. Remember that colors are a sign of high antioxidant content and other fabulous vitamins and minerals. Don't forget that Appendix B has a full guide to antioxidants!

## Unrefined Starches

When I was growing up, only one thing went into this category: lots and lots of white rice. Now, when I have white rice, I have a

---

39 "The Role of Oxalates in Autism and Chronic Disorders," The Weston A. Price Foundation, last modified March 26, 2010, accessed September 16, 2015, http://www.westonaprice.org/health-topics/the-role-of-oxalates-in-autism-and-chronic-disorders/.

few tricks to make it more flavorful and nutritious. I make white rice with some type of broth, and I love to add in seaweed. Plus, I've expanded what I eat so now there's white rice, brown rice, quinoa, sweet potatoes, and squashes. Legumes, lentils, and beans can also go into this category. You can also try buckwheat, millet, and amaranth. Explore!

# Protein

Protein is something I get asked about a lot, and I actually think protein has become too stressed in today's society. I'm a serious recreational athlete, teaching five to seven fitness/capoeira classes a week, plus doing my own capoeira training and restorative exercises; I use my body a lot. I often get questions about which protein powder is better and the timing with which to eat, and I have to admit, I don't do any of these things. What I do, however, is make sure I'm eating a nutrient-dense diet, eating when I'm hungry, and stopping when I'm satiated. Whatever makes things more simple for me is what I find works.

For the Nourished Bowl, if you are an omnivore, include different pasture-raised meats and sustainably caught fish (check out the Monterey Bay Aquarium's *Seafood Watch Guide*). If you are vegetarian, beans, lentils, and tempeh can go here.

|||||||||||||||||||||||||||||||||||||||||||||||||||||||||||||||||||||||||||||||||||||||||||||||||||||||||||||||||||||||||||||||||||

NOURISHING NOTE: A good rule of thumb is to eat about 8 grams of protein for every 20 pounds of weight. This is a minimum requirement, so those who are convalescing or pregnant may want to eat a bit more. Check out Appendix D for protein amounts in common foods.

|||||||||||||||||||||||||||||||||||||||||||||||||||||||||||||||||||||||||||||||||||||||||||||||||||||||||||||||||||||||||||||||||||

## CHAPTER 4

# 21-Day Guide to Eating Whole, Traditional Foods

In the preceding chapters, you've gotten a general overview of how to view health in a nourishing, holistic way. We've now come to the specific nourished belly guide, which should be approached slowly. You can only do so much and absorb so much information at once. I always work with my clients to add small steps one at a time; otherwise, they are bound to fall off of all the great changes they are trying to incorporate.

Also, nutritional information is also not always accurate. It's always important to read health information with a discerning eye, including what is in this book. I have tried my best to be accurate in my information, but new information comes to light every day. The most important guide you have is *how food makes*

*you feel.* (I personally do a quick test: Do I feel energized? Yes. Am I bloated? No. Success!) If you eat something and it doesn't work for you, then scrap it. Experiment to find the right lifestyle and way of eating that works for you.

Same with the recipes: Use them as a guide, but feel free to experiment! I personally use recipes as inspiration, and they can be great teachers when are you are just becoming comfortable in the kitchen. Feel free to add ingredients, and don't scrap a recipe just because you don't happen to have everything. You are *supposed* to make mistakes in the kitchen. As you work on the life skill of learning to feed yourself, making mistakes is how you learn and expand.

At the most basic logistical level, decide *when* you have time to work on your health for 21 days. The weeks before a best friend's wedding are probably not an ideal time. Find some space in your calendar where you have at least a month when you are planning on being at home and don't have too many commitments.

In this chapter, you'll learn the three levels of participation in meal planning, how to get your kitchen ready for the diet, and what basic grocery items to buy beforehand. Stocking your pantry can be pricey, so you might want to spread out your purchases over a few weeks or a month before you start the 21 days.

# Levels of Participation

The path to better eating and feeling better is a winding road, and each of us takes a different path to get there. It's important, before you decide to delve into the Nourished Belly Diet to assess where you are and to choose a level of participation that stretches you, but doesn't go over the top. You don't want to move too far, too fast, because you don't want to guarantee a crashing return back to your old habits. Choose a level that is exciting, but not overwhelming, and stick to it.

# Level 1: Baby Steps

If you've never cooked before, and this is the first time that you are attempting to make your own meals, then this is the level for you. The purpose of this level is to introduce making foods at home and beginning to create the habits of a whole foods lifestyle. Level 1's goals are:

1. Drink hot water with lemon or herbal tea when you wake up.

2. Create a weekly routine of food shopping (Where do you go? What day?).

3. Set a day where you have two hours to prepare food.

4. Make the broth of the week and the grain of the week, and buy the ferment of the week.

5. Choose at least one or two days to follow part of the meal plan. (Soup is very easy to start with and hard to make a mistake with; bringing it for lunch is a cinch!)

6. Incorporate fermented foods that you purchase at the store (sauerkraut, kimchi, yogurt).

7. Incorporate broth into your snacks and daily routine.

8. For three days each week, keep a food journal. Write down what you eat and how much, and record how you feel after eating. This is an excellent tool that I use myself and with my clients to create awareness and accountability with what we eat.

# Level 2: I Can Handle This!

If you are used to cooking a few meals a week and feel comfortable in the kitchen, then this is the right level for you. The purpose of this step is to follow the meal plan for three to four days each week, or follow most of the dinner plans. Level 2's goals are:

1. Drink herbal tea or hot water with lemon when you wake up.

2. Incorporate more herbal teas.

3. Solidify your food shopping schedule.

4. Carve out at least three to four separate days where you are following the meal plan.

5. Incorporate broth into your snacks and daily routine.

6. Incorporate fermented foods into your meals (sauerkraut, kimchi, yogurt).

7. Keep a food journal for at least three consecutive days each week.

## Level 3: Hardcore

If you feel comfortable in the kitchen and make many of your meals at home, then this is the level for you. This level will take more time, and you do need to carve out a little more time during food prep days to batch cook, but I guarantee this will feel like an accomplishment when you are done! Level 3's goals:

1. Follow the meal plan for 5 to 7 days, and snacks as well!

2. Drink hot water with lemon or herbal teas when you wake up.

3. Incorporate more herbal teas.

4. Solidify your food shopping schedule.

5. Carve out a little time each day for food prep.

6. Set two to three longer cooking sessions a week.

7. Incorporate either homemade or store-bought fermented foods.

# Setting up Your Kitchen

It is much more fun to cook in a well-stocked kitchen. In reality, you could be a master chef and make do with just a great kitchen knife, but a few gadgets go a long way. Here are some must-haves in my kitchen.

KITCHEN KNIVES: Get a 6- to 8-inch chef's knife and you'll be set for most of what you want to make in the kitchen. I've seen one too many clients try to make entire meals with a 3-inch paring knife. It takes too long! Also, make sure your knives are sharp—there's nothing more frustrating than trying to cut with dull knives. They are serious time wasters. If you have dull knives in your kitchen, it's worth getting them sharpened at your local hardware store. You can't just sharpen knives at home using the honer, which is that wand looking thing that comes with your Thanksgiving carving set. Honers keep sharp knives sharp. Don't forget to tuck in your fingers when you chop things.

**LARGE CUTTING BOARD:** Bamboo is the new, more sustainable material used to make cutting boards. You might want to have a separate cutting board for garlic and onion as the flavors tend to linger, and garlic-flavored watermelon is not my favorite thing.

**COOKWARE:** You'll mainly need a stockpot, saucepans, and sauté pans. Stay away from Teflon! It's full of chemicals that can leach into your food. I use stainless steel; cast iron is great too. If it's Christmas or your birthday, ask for an enamel-coated cast-iron pan, like Le Creuset. It's pricey, but fabulous. All in all, a good set of cookware should cost you about $250 and up; it's worth it not to get the cheapest set. One nice thing about having a cast-iron pan is that you can go from stovetop directly into the oven, which for some dishes, like The Perfect Steak recipe (page 156), is a really handy thing to do.

**SPATULA:** When you make a lot of sauces and dips, you want a spatula to scrape all that goodness out and not let anything go to waste.

**SIEVE:** This is so helpful for rinsing quinoa, draining soaked nuts, or making large batches of tea. Get a stainless steel one.

**FUNNELS:** In my kitchen, I have one that can fit into thin bottles for drinking teas, and then a larger one that fits into the mouth of my mason jars so that I can freeze and store my big pots of stews and yummy foods without making a big mess. It is a time-saver because you aren't always cleaning up after yourself, at least not so much.

**MASON JARS:** Mason jars have changed my kitchen. I do my best to steer clear of plastic, especially when storing and heating food. If you still have plastic containers for storing food, recycle them! Instead, use multipurpose mason jars; Ball jars are made in the United States! You can drink directly out of them, freeze stuff in them (don't fill them too full), and use them to transport food. They are spillproof if you screw the lids on tightly, and they save space in the fridge. They also make great decorations, come in different sizes, and are great for storing dry pantry foods. Do you need more reasons?

**HAND BLENDER (IMMERSION BLENDER):** I almost exclusively use a hand blender instead of a food processor (although grating carrots by hand can get tedious, which is why food processors are helpful) because I like the easy clean up. I use my hand blender to make pesto, hummus, soups, and the yummy Avocado Chocolate Mousse recipe on page 171. You can use it to make whipped cream as well.

**MICROPLANE:** Also called zesters, these are really good for, well, zesting. (Zest is great support for your liver!) Use them to finely grate cheese, nuts, ginger, or turmeric as well.

**COFFEE GRINDER (FOR SPICES):** I have a separate coffee grinder just for spices, and I probably use it the most for grinding my flaxseeds right before I eat them.

**ELECTRIC KETTLE:** My clients and I drink tons of herbal teas, and I have zero patience now to actually wait for a kettle to boil. Electric kettles are a huge time-saver, and they'll turn themselves off when they are ready.

**PARCHMENT PAPER:** I tend to use a lot of parchment paper in my kitchen because I dehydrate a lot of things and bake a lot of things, and I cannot for the life of me find a cookie sheet that doesn't have a Teflon coating. Teflon is that nonstick coating that has a tendency to scratch and put all sorts of yucky stuff into your food that you don't want. So, I put parchment paper over it. Then I compost the paper.

**DEHYDRATOR:** I *love* the dehydrator. Once you start soaking all your seeds, a dehydrator is a huge time-saver since you just put things in and leave them. I also use it to make granola and a lot of other yummy snacks. This is another kitchen investment, around $150 to $300, but worth it.

**SLOW COOKER:** A slow cooker is a huge lifesaver that cooks things slowly and at a low temperature. You almost can't mess up since you are cooking over a long period of time, which lets flavors gently melt into your meal. I use my slow cooker to make bone broth, braise meats, cook beans, and make soups. It's *fabulous*.

**BLENDER:** When I find myself really busy, a blender is super helpful to make power smoothies!

**WATER FILTER:** Having clean water is very important. We have a lot of stuff in our tap water that doesn't belong in our bodies. Chlorine and flouride can be very damaging. I like Multipure water systems and Berkey systems. Another investment, this will cost you around $300 to $400, but considering the amount of water you should be drinking, it's worth it.

## Pantry Makeover

How does your pantry look? I've been working on my pantry for a while, with the aim that when things get really busy, I won't have tempting, degenerative foods at arms reach and will have a store of regenerative, whole foods that I can pull from to make a quick and fantastic meal. Pantry items are meant to be shelf stable, at least if stored in the right conditions (usually out of direct sunlight or in a dark, cool place). They are there for you when you need them.

Step one would be to clean out what's in your pantry that is either super old (if you don't remember when you bought it, compost it) or degenerative. You want your pantry to support your healthy lifestyle.

Below, you'll find some suggestions of great pantry items that you'll need if you are following the 21-day guide, and if you don't get around to using them now, you can use them on a later date. If you buy these all at once, they put a little dent into your pocketbook, so perhaps spreading these purchases out over a period of time will be helpful.

The fats, oils, and nuts list is a starter kit to healthy fats in your pantry. Some oils are delicate and are degraded when exposed to heat and light, so it's better to store things in a dark, cool place. I personally put nuts in the freezer until I'm about to use them.

For grains and starches, purchase ½ to 1 pound at a time.

| Fats, Oils, and Nuts | Grains/Starches | Herbs/Spices | Miscellaneous |
|---|---|---|---|
| Almonds | Brown rice | Bay leaves | Apple cider vinegar |
| Butter | Millet | Cinnamon | |
| Cashews | Oats | Cocoa powder | Baking soda |
| Chia seeds (no need for cold storage, a cool place is fine) | Quinoa | Coriander seed | Coconut milk (I like Native Forest Brand) |
| | Winter squash (your choice) | Cumin | |
| | Sweet potatoes | Garam masala | Dates |
| Coconut oil | | Rosemary | Maple syrup |
| Flaxseeds (no need for cold storage, a cool place is fine) | **Proteins** | Sea salt | Miso (white) |
| | | Star anise | |
| Peanut butter or other nut butter | Black beans | Turmeric | Nori sheets |
| | | Vanilla | Organic corn tortillas |
| Pumpkin seeds | Canned fish (e.g., sardines or wild salmon) | | Seaweed (kombu, wakame) |
| Sunflower seeds | | | |
| Tahini | Lentils (red and green) | **Liquids** | Vermicelli noodles |
| Toasted sesame seed oil | | | |
| | | Filtered water (use lemons and limes for flavoring) | |
| | | Green tea | |
| | | Herbal teas (mint, nettle, dandelion root, rooibos) | |

# Preparing a Place to Eat

Most of us eat on the run, in front of the TV, or in front of our computers. When you don't stop to slow down, your body is still in go mode, and your digestion doesn't switch on. There's a reason nutrition and health professional like to quote the popular saying, "Rest and digest."

How do you eat every day? Do you usually sit down in front of the TV or keep working through lunch? If yes, then how can you structure your mealtimes to support digestion and actually let your mind take a break?

Next time you eat, turn off your electronics, and find a beautiful place to enjoy your meal. Take the time to think about chewing carefully. I've read suggestions that say to chew your food 30 times, which I find pretty difficult. I say chew so that everything is chewed. Don't swallow things whole! When you are done, go back to what you were doing. Your body and brain will thank you.

## CHAPTER 5

# Weekly Meal Plans

You are about to get started on your weekly meal plans—exciting! That's why you are here. Don't forget, there are three different levels you can choose from. If ever you cannot find a specific ingredient, feel free to substitute.

Each level will also focus on a broth of the week, grain of the week, and ferment of the week. The broth should be started on Saturday morning or night. The broth and grain can be used as desired for any of your meals, and think of the ferment as a fun thing to try.

Every week, take advantage of the Weekly Planner, which is a large part of being successful on this plan. Figure out which days you'll go grocery shopping, make lists of ingredients you'll need, and reflect on what has gone well from the week before. There is also the option of working on a lifestyle habit from the holistic health assessment (page 26).

Remember for all levels:

- Drink half your weight in ounces each day; this can be a combo of water, herbal teas, and broth.

- First thing in the morning, drink 1 cup of warm water with lemon or herbal tea.

Here's a refresher on the levels:

## Level 1: Baby Steps

If you are in the first level, you are not feeling so comfortable in the kitchen, and your job in these next three weeks is to make a few of the basics. Each week you'll try a different broth and choose one to two days to do some cooking. You decide which recipes you'd like to make. You can buy the suggested ferment of the week and try it out in one of your meals. By the end of the three weeks, you should feel comfortable making soups and broths, and be able to make a few basics. This is a great start to getting in the kitchen!

## Level 2: I Can Handle This!

As a Level 2, you are comfortable in the kitchen, but due to falling out of the habit or maybe lacking inspiration, you have gotten used to eating out and perhaps indulging a bit too much. Level 2s should make the broth of the week and choose three to four days to cook. By the end of the three weeks, you should continue the habit of cooking a few days a week and making broth a part of your weekly routine.

## Level 3: Hardcore

Level 3s feel comfortable in the kitchen and are perhaps making quite a few meals at home. However, you may just need an extra push to really cut out processed foods and eat as cleanly as possible. Level 3s commit to spending the most time in the kitchen. For you, the next 21 days are about focusing on eating a clean, whole foods diet. The more days you choose to cook at home the better, but choose anywhere between five to seven days to eat meals that you make at home. At the end of the next 21 days, since you will only be nourishing your body with whole foods, you should feel in tip-top shape.

Okay, make sense? Remember, this is an exploration that you can come back to and modify again and again. I do suggest that at some point, whether it simply be for one week or three, when you are ready, go hardcore! You will feel a world of difference when you are ONLY putting whole foods into your body.

# Week 1

All levels make the broth, grain, and ferment of the week. Use them as desired in your weekly meal plan.

## Broth of the Week: Chicken Broth

When I first introduce bone broth to clients, I often start with chicken. Our society seems to be less squeamish around chicken bones than beef or lamb bones. I get it. I either make my chicken broth with an entire chicken carcass, or I save bones in my freezer when I buy chicken legs or drumsticks, and when I have a good pile, I make a broth.

Chicken bones make a wonderful go-to broth. I almost always have a jar of chicken broth in my fridge ready to go! I recommend leaving chicken bones in the slow cooker for at least 15 hours; I leave mine for around 36 hours.

## Grain of the Week: Quinoa

If you've never made quinoa before, then you must try this! I eat more quinoa than I do brown rice, and it goes with absolutely everything. It's high in protein, low in starch, and packed with vitamins. For those who are going gluten free, quinoa is a great, delicious option to replace pasta and bread. You can cook it plain with just quinoa and water or broth, or check out the Mushroom Garlic Quinoa recipe on page 92 for a little extra flavor.

# Ferment of the Week: Miso

Most of you know miso from the soup that you get before you eat sushi, yes? Miso is so much more than just soup. It contains glutamates that enhance flavor, provides a dose of healthy beneficial bacteria, and is great as a marinade and in salad dressings. Miso is a fermented paste made up of soybeans, a bacteria starter, salt, and a grain, usually rice or barley.

In general, I'm not a large advocate of soy since its proteins can be hard to digest, but one of the few ways that I encourage my clients to eat soy is in the form of miso. The fermenting process helps to break down some of the long, hard-to-digest proteins and isoflavones.

There are many different kinds; some can be more savory and some can be sweeter. White miso is generally milder and is a nice form to ease yourself into. Always buy organic, as conventional soy is genetically modified.

My mother marinates fish in miso or uses it as a glaze for meats. I generally like to apply miso at the end of the cooking process to preserve the bacteria. High heating of miso destroys some of its beneficial qualities, so using it as a dressing is a wonderful way to add it into your diet knowing that all the bacteria are alive and kicking!

## Suggested Menu, Week 1

LEVEL 1: Choose one to two cooking days.

LEVEL 2: Choose three to four cooking days.

LEVEL 3: Choose five to seven cooking days.

| Week 1 | | |
|---|---|---|
| **SATURDAY** | **Morning prep** | Make Whole Chicken Broth (page 88). |
| | **Breakfast** | 1 cup Sweet Millet Cereal (page 111)<br>1 cup nettle tea |
| | **Lunch** | 3 ounces (palm size) The Perfect Steak (page 156)<br>1 cup Garlic Cauliflower Mash (page 138)<br>1 cup Bok Choy, Mushrooms, and Garlic (page 133) |
| | **Snack** | Veggie sticks<br>1 cup dandelion root tea |
| | **Dinner** | 1 cup Massaged Chicken and Kale Salad with Honey Miso Dressing (page 128)<br>3 ounces marinated steak strips from leftovers of The Perfect Steak |
| **SUNDAY** | **Breakfast** | ½ cup leftover Garlic Cauliflower Mash<br>1–2 fried eggs<br>1 cup Bacon and Collards (page 134) |
| | **Lunch** | 1 cup Aloo Gobi (page 140)<br>½ cup Mushroom Garlic Quinoa (page 92)<br>1 cup leftover chicken from Whole Chicken Broth |
| | **Snack** | 1 cup Whole Chicken Broth, salted, to taste |
| | **Dinner** | 1 cup leftover Bacon and Collards<br>½–1 cup leftover chicken from Whole Chicken Broth mixed with 2 tablespoons Seasonal Pumpkin Seed Pesto (page 123)<br>1 cup Cashew Milk Shake (page 176) |
| | **Night prep** | Make Quinoa Bites (page 116) for the morning. |
| **MONDAY** | **Breakfast** | 2–3 Quinoa Bites<br>1 cup green tea |
| | **Lunch** | 1 cup leftover Aloo Gobi<br>½ cup quinoa with 2 tablespoons minced cilantro or green herb |
| | **Snack** | Leftover Cashew Milk Shake |
| | **Dinner** | 1 cup Coconut Red Lentils (page 150)<br>½ cup leftover Mushroom Garlic Quinoa<br>1 cup sautéed kale |

| | | |
|---|---|---|
| **TUESDAY** | **Breakfast** | 1 cup whole plain yogurt<br>1 cup seasonal fruit |
| | **Lunch** | 1 cup leftover Coconut Red Lentils<br>½ cup leftover Mushroom Garlic Quinoa<br>1 cup sautéed kale |
| | **Snack** | 1 cup Whole Chicken Broth with coconut milk, lemon juice, and salt, to taste |
| | **Dinner** | 1½ cups Chicken Miso Soup (page 162)<br>½ cup leftover Mushroom Garlic Quinoa |
| **WEDNESDAY** | **Breakfast** | 1 cup leftover Aloo Gobi<br>1 tablespoon whole plain yogurt with 2 tablespoons minced cilantro, to garnish |
| | **Lunch** | 2–3 Chicken Curry Collard Wraps (page 159) |
| | **Snack** | 1 cup herbal tea<br>1 piece seasonal fruit |
| | **Dinner** | 3 ounces Miso-Glazed Dover Sole (page 166)<br>1 cup Coconut Kale (page 139)<br>½ cup quinoa |
| **THURSDAY** | **Breakfast** | 1½ cups leftover Miso Chicken Soup |
| | **Lunch** | 1½ cups Vermicelli Noodle Soup (page 161)<br>3 ounces leftover Miso-Glazed Dover Sole |
| | **Snack** | 1–2 leftover Quinoa Bites |
| | **Dinner** | 3–4 Taiwanese Tacos (page 164)<br>1 cup sautéed cauliflower |
| **FRIDAY** | You are on your own today! Look at the leftovers you have and plan what you'd like to eat. | |

# Week 2

All levels make the broth, grain, and ferment of the week. Use them as desired in your weekly meal plan.

## Broth of the Week: Beef Broth

Beef broth is used around the world, from Taiwanese beef noodle soup to Eastern European borscht to Mexican *caldo de res*. All of these delicious, traditional stews use beef broth as the starting component. It's delicious, nourishing, and extremely comforting.

This week, you will focus on making soups and stews from beef broth. See page 87 for the recipe. Remember beef bones are heartier and you can simmer beef bones for up to 48 hours. You can even make two separate batches from the same bones. I often take out the broth after 24 hours and put in more filtered water for another 24. It is one of the stronger broths that you can make; some people find the flavor a little overpowering, but I like it!

## Grain of the Week: Brown Rice

Oh, rice! I have such a long history with you! In Taiwanese, the word for "meal" is actually "rice." "Did you eat rice yet?" people ask when you greet them. Rice has a special place in my heart; as a child, one of my favorite things to eat was a forkful of warm rice straight from the rice cooker.

The most common types of rice are short grain and long grain, which can be either white or brown. This week, you will focus on cooking with brown rice, which contains way more nutrients than white rice since the outer nutritious bran is not removed. This outer bran contains pretty much everything important: proteins, vitamin E, vitamin B complex, and starch. I also really like the flavor of brown rice. See page 90 for the recipe.

# Ferment of the Week: Sauerkraut

If you haven't played around with eating sauerkrauts, take this week to do so! Either buy some unpasteurized sauerkrauts at the store (pasteurization kills the beneficial bacteria that we are trying to keep alive), or try your hand at making some yourself (see page 98). I would suggest buying some so you can get the benefits right away, and then if you have time this week, try making a batch. It won't be ready for a few weeks anyway, so see what happens!

## Suggested Menu, Week 2

**LEVEL 1:** Choose one to two cooking days.

**LEVEL 2:** Choose three to four cooking days.

**LEVEL 3:** Choose five to seven cooking days.

| | Week 2 | |
|---|---|---|
| | **Morning prep** | Make Beef Bone Broth (page 87). |
| | **Breakfast** | 1 cup Savory Oatmeal (page 113) |
| | | 1 cup green tea |
| | **Lunch** | 4 ounces Roasted Rosemary Chicken Legs (page 157) |
| SATURDAY | | 1 cup Roasted Brussels Sprouts and Bacon (page 137) or seasonal veggies |
| | | ½ cup Brown Rice (page 90) |
| | **Snack** | 1 cup whole plain yogurt |
| | | 1 cup seasonal fruit |
| | **Dinner** | ½ cup Homestyle Ground Beef (page 152) |
| | | ½ cup Brown Rice |
| | | 1 cup sautéed broccoli and garlic |
| | | 2 tablespoons Sauerkraut (page 98) |

| | | |
|---|---|---|
| **SUNDAY** | **Breakfast** | 1 cup Hearty Rice Porridge (page 118)<br>1 fried egg<br>1 cup leftover roasted Brussel Sprouts and Bacon<br>¼ cup Sauerkraut<br>1 cup nettle tea |
| | **Lunch** | 1½ cups Sausage Lentil Broccoli Soup (page 147)<br>½ cup Brown Rice<br>1 cup sautéed spinach and garlic |
| | **Snack** | Veggie sticks with 2 tablespoons Tahini Miso Dressing (page 124) |
| | **Dinner** | 1 cup Massaged Chicken and Kale Salad with Honey Miso Dressing (page 128)<br>½ cup leftover Roasted Rosemary Chicken Legs<br>2 tablespoons leftover Tahini Miso Dressing<br>½ cup Avocado Chocolate Mousse (page 171) |
| **MONDAY** | **Breakfast** | 1 cup Power Smoothie (page 114)<br>1 cup green tea |
| | **Lunch** | 1 cup leftover Sausage Lentil Broccoli Soup<br>½ cup Brown Rice<br>1 cup sautéed kale drizzled with lemon juice, extra virgin olive oil, and salt, to taste<br>2 tablespoons Sauerkraut |
| | **Snack** | Banana with nut butter |
| | **Dinner** | 3 ounces Lemon Salmon (page 167)<br>½ cup Brown Rice<br>1 cup sautéed broccoli and cauliflower with garlic |

| | | |
|---|---|---|
| **TUESDAY** | **Breakfast** | 1 cup leftover Hearty Rice Porridge with 1 cup spinach mixed in while reheating<br><br>3 ounces leftover Lemon Salmon<br><br>1 cup mint tea |
| | **Lunch** | ½ cup Homestyle Ground Beef garnished with 2 tablespoons whole plain yogurt<br><br>½ cup Brown Rice<br><br>1 cup leftover sautéed broccoli and cauliflower with garlic |
| | **Snack** | 1–2 hard-boiled eggs with ½ avocado and pesto |
| | **Dinner** | 3 ounces pork chop<br><br>½ cup Homestyle Black Beans (page 148)<br><br>1 cup roasted squash<br><br>1 cup sautéed kale with garlic |
| **WEDNESDAY** | **Breakfast** | 1–2 fried eggs<br><br>1 cup leftover Homestyle Black Beans and rice<br><br>¼ cup loosely chopped cilantro<br><br>2 tablespoons Sauerkraut |
| | **Lunch** | 1 cup leftover Sausage Lentil Broccoli Soup<br><br>½ cup Brown Rice<br><br>½ cup leftover roasted squash |
| | **Snack** | 1 cup whole plain yogurt<br><br>1 cup seasonal fruit<br><br>1 teaspoon chia seeds<br><br>Handful of nuts |
| | **Dinner** | 1½ cups Peanut Oxtail Stew (page 153) or Comforting Russian Borscht (page 154) |

| | | |
|---|---|---|
| **THURSDAY** | **Breakfast** | 1 cup Power Oatmeal (page 112)<br>1 cup nettle tea |
| | **Lunch** | 1½ cups leftover Peanut Oxtail Stew or Comforting Russian Borscht |
| | **Snack** | Hard-boiled egg with Seasonal Pumpkin Seed Pesto (page 123) |
| | **Dinner** | 3 ounces leftover pork chop<br>1 cup leftover Homestyle Black Beans and rice<br>1 cup steamed kale |
| | **Night Prep** | Look at your leftovers, and plan for Friday, because you are on your own then! |
| **FRIDAY** | | You are on your own today! Look at the leftovers you have and plan what you'd like to eat. |

# Week 3

All levels make the broth, grain, and ferment of the week. Use them as desired in your weekly meal plan.

## Broth of the Week: Veggie Broth

Veggie broth is a beautiful way to use leftover veggie scraps and to drink some mineral-rich broth. I like to keep some in my thermos throughout the day, and for those of my clients who are vegetarian, veggie broth is a great substitute for bone broth as a nutritious beverage.

I save my veggie scraps in the freezer and add them to a few whole vegetables to be thrifty and get a nice, well-rounded flavor.

## Grain of the Week: Polenta

Many ancient cultures used corn as a staple, and the US carries on the tradition. Corn is one of the most widely grown crops in the US, and corn by-products are ubiquitous in processed foods and industrial goods. The use of corn is part of a larger conversation about food policy, but the variety that graces our tables is a long-time comfort food! One of the ways in which I eat corn is in the form of polenta. I love to introduce polenta to clients because it's a simple way to create a very quick meal as it stores well and is pretty darn versatile. (See Creamy Polenta recipe on page 93.)

## Ferment of the Week: Kombucha

I don't drink kombucha all the time because it can be rather sweet, but once in a while, it's a really nice addition to my day.

# Suggested Menu, Week 3

LEVEL 1: Choose one to two cooking days.

LEVEL 2: Choose three to four cooking days.

LEVEL 3: Choose five to seven cooking days.

| | | Week 3 |
|---|---|---|
| **SATURDAY** | **Morning prep** | Make Veggie Mineral Broth (page 89). |
| | **Breakfast** | Huevos Pericos (page 120)<br>2 corn tortillas<br>1 tablespoon chopped chives (or any green herb), to garnish |
| | **Lunch** | 1 cup seasonal veggie dish, such as Eggplant and Peppers with Cashew Garlic Cream (page 136) or Bok Choy, Mushrooms, and Garlic (page 133)<br>2 fried eggs |
| | **Snack** | ¼ cup Chicken Liver Paté (page 108)<br>1 cup carrots |
| | **Dinner** | 3 ounces The Perfect Lamb Chop (page 156)<br>1 small baked sweet potato<br>1 cup broccoli and cauliflower with garlic<br>1 cup Date Almond Milk (page 177) |
| **SUNDAY** | **Morning prep** | Place pork ribs into the slow cooker for Slow-Cooked Pork Ribs (page 165). |
| | **Breakfast** | 2–3 Coconut Banana Squash Pancakes (page 115)<br>½ cup plain whole yogurt<br>2 strips bacon |
| | **Lunch** | 1½ cups Kabocha Squash and Coconut Soup (page 163)<br>3 ounces leftovers The Perfect Lamb Chop, garnished with 2 tablespoons cilantro |
| | **Snack** | 1 cup fruit with nut butter<br>1 cup Veggie Broth with sea salt, to taste |
| | **Dinner** | 2–3 Slow-Cooked Pork Ribs<br>1 cup Creamy Polenta (page 93)<br>2 tablespoons Cashew Garlic Cream (page 125)<br>1 cup sautéed collard greens |

| | | |
|---|---|---|
| **MONDAY** | **Breakfast** | 1 cup Savory Oatmeal (page 113)<br>2 tablespoons leftover Cashew Garlic Cream |
| | **Lunch** | 2 Sardine Nori Wraps (page 104) |
| | **Snack** | ¼ cup leftover Chicken Liver Paté<br>Handful of carrot sticks |
| | **Dinner** | 2 leftover Slow-Cooked Pork Ribs<br>2 corn tortillas<br>1 cup leftover Kabocha Squash and Coconut Soup<br>1 cup sautéed broccoli with bacon |
| **TUESDAY** | **Breakfast** | ½ cup leftover Creamy Polenta<br>1–2 fried eggs<br>1 cup sautéed cauliflower<br>1 tablespoon chives, to garnish |
| | **Lunch** | 2 leftover Slow-Cooked Pork Ribs<br>1 cup sautéed kale<br>1 sweet potato with 1 tablespoon butter |
| | **Snack** | 1 cup Veggie Broth with sea salt, to taste |
| | **Dinner** | 2 cups Salmon Stew (page 168) |
| **WEDNESDAY** | **Breakfast** | 2 cups leftover Salmon Stew |
| | **Lunch** | 1½ cups leftover Kabocha Squash and Coconut Soup<br>1 cup sautéed collard greens |
| | **Snack** | 1 cup Seasonal Fruit Parfait (page 109) |
| | **Dinner** | 1 cup Garlic Shrimp (page 169)<br>2 strips bacon<br>½ cup leftover Creamy Polenta<br>2 tablespoons leftover Garlic Cashew Cream<br>1 cup sautéed kale |

 *The* Nourished Belly Diet

| | | |
|---|---|---|
| **THURSDAY** | **Breakfast** | 1 cup Savory Oatmeal<br>½ cup leftover Garlic Shrimp |
| | **Lunch** | 2 cups leftover Salmon Stew |
| | **Snack** | Handful of carrot sticks<br>½ cup leftover Chicken Liver Paté |
| | **Dinner** | 1 cup leftover Kabocha Squash and Coconut Soup<br>1 cup sautéed spinach<br>2–3 slices Baked Portobellos (page 145) |
| **FRIDAY** | | You are on your own today! Look at the leftovers you have and plan what you'd like to eat. |

# Weekly Action Planner

Okay, you've got the suggested meal plans. Now, the level you'd like to participate in is up to you. Choose something that will stretch you, not overwhelm you. Figure out which days you'll grocery shop, which days you'll cook, and what ingredients you'll need. Also assess your weekly progress. Ask yourself:

- What went well from the previous week?

- What did you learn?

- What were some challenges?

# Action Steps

| | Action Steps |
|---|---|
| Saturday | |
| Sunday | |
| Monday | |
| Tuesday | |
| Wednesday | |
| Thursday | |
| Friday | |

*Blank copies of this planner can be found at www.TheNourishedBelly.com.

## Lifestyle Habits

Are there additional lifestyle habits you would like to work on, such as drinking more water, or going to sleep earlier? Choose one each week that you'd like to expand on.

## CHAPTER 6

# Recipes

In the following chapter, you'll find all of my favorite recipes I make to nourish myself and others. I've included a more detailed section on all the ins and outs of nourishing cooking in Chapter 7, Holistic Nutrition 101, including the bioavailability of foods, cooked versus raw foods, and the basics of making a delicious meal!

# The Basics

Where do you start? Here, at the basics! I think the first thing I learned to cook were scrambled eggs (and I've only recently perfected this technique). I also recall sautéing a bunch of broccoli. Remember, whatever it is that you start with, it's a trial run. Cooking is always an experiment, and once you get the hang of it, the experiments will usually turn out amazing.

Think about what you want to start with first. Maybe making a grain or a bone broth. Both are easy and delicious. Whatever you do, be forgiving if it doesn't turn out, and try again! You'll get the hang of it. Have fun!

# Cooking Meat

||||||||||||||||||||||||||||||||||||||||||||||||||||||||||||||||||||||||||||||||||||||||||||||||||||||||||||||||||||||||||||||||||||||||||

I didn't cook meat for a long time because every time I tried, I just couldn't get it right. I would spend a chunk of change to buy a beautiful piece of meat, then it would just come out too tough, too dry, and unenjoyable. Buzz kill.

Finally, I took some cooking lessons and learned what actually happens to animal protein when you cook it. There's a science behind it. It's complicated, however, since different cuts of meat have different properties. Generally, however, this is what happens:

STAGE 1: When you start to cook the meat, and it reaches a temperature of around 120°F, there is an initial coming together of molecules, and water is squeezed out of cells into the meat. This is when meat is served rare and is juicy and tender.

STAGE 2: As the meat reaches 140°F, proteins come together and juices are released from the meat, making the cut shrink and become tougher and chewier. (This is the stage that I often mistakenly got to.)

STAGE 3: As you continue to cook meat to around 160°F, the collagen breaks down and coats the muscle fibers, giving the meat a succulent texture.

What should you do then?

FOR SINGLE CUTS (5-8 OUNCES) OF LAMB, PORK, BEEF, AND CHICKEN:

1. Sprinkle each side of the meat with salt before cooking.

2. Take an ovensafe pan, put it on high heat on the stovetop with a little oil, and sear the meat on the outside until lightly brown. About 2 minutes per side.

3. Finish the meat at lower temperature like 300°F, for roughly 5–7 minutes.

4. Take the meat out of the oven just before it's done and let it sit. It will finish cooking on its own.

Look at The Perfect Steak recipe on page 156 for a slightly different method. See which one you like best!

FOR LARGER (1-2 POUNDS) CUTS LIKE LONDON BROIL, PORK BUTT, SHANKS, AND PORK BELLY:

1. Salt and brown. (You can skip the browning part if you're short on time.)

2. Put it in the slow cooker with a bit of broth, and let it cook for the day.

# Bone Broth

Bone broth is super simple to make. Trust me! Sometimes it takes time to figure out where to buy bones (most local grocery stores and farmers markets will have bones), but once you do it, it's easy.

**MAKES ROUGHLY 3–4 QUARTS**

1-2 pounds bones (You can mix bones, but I usually keep my chicken bones separate since the flavors can be different.)

2 tablespoons apple cider vinegar

1 medium yellow onion, roughly chopped

4 carrots, including tops, roughly chopped

4 stalks celery, roughly chopped

2 bay leaves

1.  Place the bones at the bottom of a stockpot or slow cooker, covering the bones with filtered water.

2.  Add the apple cider vinegar. The vinegar will help to pull the minerals from the bones.

3.  Bring the broth to a boil and then reduce to a simmer.

4.  Bones should be easily crushed—this means you've extracted as much as you can out of them! Follow these cooking times:

- Fish: no more than 6 hours (keep the fish heads!)
- Chicken: 12–24 hours
- Lamb and goat: 36 hours
- Pork and beef: 36–48 hours

5.  For the last 4 hours of cooking, add the onion, carrots, celery, and any other vegetables of your choosing, along with the bay leaves. Using a strainer, funnel the broth into jars. Freeze some (label with the date and kind of broth) and keep some in the fridge for immediate use!

You can definitely cook broth on the stovetop, but sometimes this can backfire, since you can forget about it and leave the house! (Which I've done.) Some people leave the broth on all day, turn it off at night, and then simmer again in the morning. I prefer to use a slow cooker so I can just put the bones in and forget about it until it's done.

# Whole Chicken Broth

||||||||||||||||||||||||||||||||||||||||||||||||||||||||||||||||||||||||||||||||||||||||||||||||||||

MAKES 4 QUARTS

1 whole chicken

4 quarts water, divided

2 tablespoons apple cider vinegar

1 medium yellow onion

4 medium carrots

4 stalks celery

2 bay leaves

1. Place whole chicken into stockpot or slow cooker.

2. Cover completely with the first 2 quarts of water and add the apple cider vinegar.

3. Simmer for 4–6 hours.

4. Take out the chicken and pull meat from bones. Careful, it's hot!

5. Store meat in the fridge for use throughout the week.

6. Place the bones back into broth, and place the remaining 2 quarts of water in.

7. Simmer for another 12–24 hours. In the last 4 hours, add the onion, carrots, celery, and bay leaves.

8. Strain and store in glass jars.

# Veggie Mineral Broth

Making a great veggie broth is simple, nutritious, and hydrating. It's full of minerals from all of those yummy vegetables that you put in, and since most of us are mineral deficient (from our poor diets and the poor soil quality), it's a great way to start adding minerals to our diets.

I love to have a cup in the morning first thing when I wake up. Or, I'll often bring a thermos with me if I'm at the office all day or out for a picnic.

Save your veggie scraps! Kale stems, pepper tops, the ends of your asparagus, corn cobs, carrot tops. Anything and everything. Keep everything in a bag in the freezer until you get about 3-4 loosely packed cups.

MAKES 2–3 QUARTS

| | |
|---|---|
| 1 onion | 1–2 sweet potatoes |
| 2–3 medium to large carrots | 1 winter squash |
| 3–4 celery stalks | 1 cup mushrooms (any kind) |
| 2–3 quarts filtered water | handful of whole seaweed |
| Optional ingredients: | 1 bunch kale |
| 3–4 cups veggie scraps (optional) | |

1. Throw everything into a stockpot or slow cooker.

2. Simmer for 3–4 hours.

3. Strain, and store! Freeze some in mason jars (don't fill the jars too full!), and put some in the fridge for use in the next 4 or 5 days.

4. Use it for making grains and stir-fries, or just having a cup with a little salt as a snack.

# Cooking Grains

||||||||||||||||||||||||||||||||||||||||||||||||||||||||||||||||||||||||||||||||||||||||||||||

Nowadays, many people avoid grains like the plague. In my view, *whole* grains can have a healthy place in the diet, and unless you have a sensitivity to certain grains, you don't need to avoid them completely. They are full of vitamins and minerals and can be part of nourishing diet.

2 cups grain

Roughly 2 cups bone broth, veggie broth, or water (Check grain-to-liquid ratio in the following table for exact amount depending on grain.)

1 tablespoon apple cider vinegar

1.  Soak your choice of grain in the liquid and 1 tablespoon of apple cider vinegar overnight. Drain.

2.  Place in a medium pot with grain and the appropriate amount of liquid.

3.  Bring to a simmer.

4.  Cover with a lid while cooking and avoid constantly checking. Check the amount of moisture left toward the last 10 minutes of cooking. Most of the liquid should have cooked off and it should look moist, not dry. When most of the liquid is gone, turn off the heat and let sit for at least 10 minutes.

||||||||||||||||||||||||||||||||||||||||||||||||||||||||||||||||||||||||||||||||||||||||||||||

NOURISHING NOTE: For the Nourished Belly Diet, you can add ½ cup of cooked grain to any soup or stew.

||||||||||||||||||||||||||||||||||||||||||||||||||||||||||||||||||||||||||||||||||||||||||||||

| Cooking Times and Yields | | | |
|---|---|---|---|
| Grain | Cook Time | Grain to Liquid Ratio | Yield for 1 dry cup |
| **Amaranth** | 20 minutes | 1:2½ | 2½ cups |
| **Barley (contains gluten)** | 35–40 minutes | 1:3 | 3 cups |
| **Brown Rice** | 40 minutes | 1:2 | 4 cups |
| **Buckwheat** | 20 minutes | 1:2 | 2 cups |
| **Millet** | 15–20 minutes | 1:2 | 3 cups |
| **Oats (rolled)** | 10 minutes | 1:2 | 1½ cups |
| **Oats (steel cut)** | 25 minutes | 1:3 | 2 cups |
| **Polenta** | 5 minutes (needs to be stirred) | 1:4 | 3 cups |
| **Quinoa** | 15–20 minutes | 1:2 | 3 cups |

# Mushroom Garlic Quinoa

||||||||||||||||||||||||||||||||||||||||||||||||||||||||||||||||||||||||||||||||||||||||||||||||||||||||||||||||

SERVES 6–8

1 large pat organic butter/coconut oil/ghee

1 small yellow onion, chopped

1 cup mushrooms (any kind), chopped

2 cloves garlic, chopped

1–2 cups rinsed quinoa

2–4 cups filtered water

1.  Place a medium to large saucepan on the stove over medium heat.

2.  Drop in the pat of butter/coconut oil/ghee.

3.  Toss in onion, mushrooms, and garlic, and stir occasionally for about 4 minutes. If onion begins to burn, turn down heat, and add a splash of water or broth.

4.  When the onion is translucent, add the quinoa and stir.

5.  Add water, cover with a lid, and simmer for approximately 20 minutes.

6.  Turn off heat and leave with lid on for roughly 10 minutes.

7.  Serve or store for later in the week. Great for scrambles and for adding ½ cup to your soup or stew.

# Creamy Polenta

When I discovered how easy and delicious polenta is to make, this quickly became part of my grain rotation. When it's polenta week, you'll be sure that some type of seafood makes it into the meal planning, as well as the Cashew Garlic Cream (page 125) and a nice, large pat of butter. Have fun with this one!

MAKES 4 CUPS

2½ cups veggie or bone broth

1½ cups milk or coconut milk

1 teaspoon salt

1 cup polenta

1. Bring liquids and salt to a boil in a medium saucepan. Slowly stir in polenta.

2. Simmer for roughly 15 minutes and stir frequently to keep polenta from sticking to the bottom.

3. Remove from heat and serve or store. You can spread the polenta onto a cookie sheet and wait until it is cooled to cut into squares and either freeze or put in the fridge.

4. Reheat by simply frying the cuts, or add more liquid until you have the consistency you want.

# Perfect Eggs

IIIIIIIIIIIIIIIIIIIIIIIIIIIIIIIIIIIIIIIIIIIIIIIIIIIIIIIIIIIIIIIIIIIIIIIIIIIIIIIIIIIIIIIIIIIIIIIIIIIIIIII

Eggs are one of the most bioavailable proteins out there. They are peppered throughout the 21-day Nourished Belly Diet. Eggs are extremely nutritious, and remember from Chapter 3's section on Healthy Fats (page 44), we aren't as concerned with dietary cholesterol like we used to be. However, be mindful of any unusual symptoms bafter you eat them, because eggs are one of the more common allergens.

FOR BOILED EGGS:

1. Place the eggs in a small saucepan with the cold water.

2. Bring to a boil, turn off heat, and let sit for the following times:

   • Softboiled: 6 minutes

   • Hardboiled: 10 minutes

3. Let stand in cool water for 5 minutes before enjoying!

FOR SCRAMBLED EGGS:

1–2 eggs

splash of cream or milk (optional)

1 tablespoon cooking oil

1. Crack each egg on a flat surface and put it in a small mixing bowl. (If shells fall in, use the half shell to scoop it out. Shell attracts shell!)

2. Add in cream or milk if desired.

3. Wisk the eggs for about 30 seconds with a fork until all parts are mixed thoroughly.

4. Heat sauté pan on medium until warm/hot.

5. Pour in the cooking oil.

6. Pour the eggs into the pan and let cook for 30 seconds.

7. Turn off the heat.

8. Using a spatula, flip and scramble the eggs until they reach the desired doness.

9. Serve.

FOR FRIED EGGS:
1 tablespoon cooking oil

2 eggs

1. Heat sauté pan on medium until warm/hot. Turn heat to low.

2. Pour in the cooking oil.

3. Crack eggs into pan.

4. Cook for 1–2 minutes.

5. Using a spatula, flip and allow to cook for 20 more seconds, or until they reach the desired runniness.

# Simple Vegetable Sauté

||||||||||||||||||||||||||||||||||||||||||||||||||||||||||||||||||||||||||||||||||||||||||||||||||||||||

Veggies play a *very* important part of the Nourished Belly equation. You have the leafy greens, such as collards, spinach, chard, and kale, then you have other colorful veggies that are often crunchy, such as broccoli, summer squash, cabbage, and carrots. Let's look at the basic recipe for a veggie sauté. Veggies should take up half of every meal, plus they are just so yummy and vibrant.

FOR LEAFY GREENS:

SERVES 2–3

spoonful of coconut oil, butter, or bacon fat

1 bunch leafy greens, roughly chopped

splash of water or broth

2 cloves garlic, minced or chopped

pinch of sea salt

1. Heat a medium sauté pan on medium heat, and add in the coconut oil, butter, or bacon fat

2. Add in greens and stir for 1 minute.

3. Add in the water or broth, and add the garlic.

4. Spinach, chard and beet greens will cook in roughly 2 minutes; transfer them out of the pan once they have changed color and wilted. Kale and collards can be sautéed for 3 minutes and covered for 1 to 2 minutes.

5. Sprinkle with sea salt and serve.

---

Tip: With heartier leafy greens, such as collards or kale, take out the stem by pinching the end of the stalk and pulling the leaf off. Save the stalks to juice or to use for broth.

---

## FOR COLORFUL, CRUNCHY VEGGIES:

**SERVES 2**

When you cook vegetables, it's helpful to look at their consistency (for example, summer squash is more spongy and will cook quicker than, say, broccoli or cabbage). You'll want to put veggies that take longer to cook in first, adding vegetables that don't need as much time as you cook. In a simple veggie stir-fry, I usually start with onions and mushrooms, add firmer veggies such as carrots and broccoli, and finish with a leafy green in the last few minutes.

Basically, you want to cut veggies into roughly the same size and shape so that they will cook at roughly the same time. You can omit the garlic if you like, but I grew up eating garlic in *everything*, so this is how I roll.

½ tablespoon cooking oil

2 cups colorful, crunchy vegetables, chopped and/or sliced

1–2 cloves garlic, minced (optional)

splash of broth or water

sea salt and pepper, to taste

1. Heat sauté pan over medium until warm.

2. Add cooking oil.

3. Add veggies, and stir until coated.

4. Add garlic if using, and stir.

5. Add splash of broth or water and cover with a lid.

6. Cook for a few minutes and taste for doneness!

7. Add salt and pepper.

# Sauerkraut

||||||||||||||||||||||||||||||||||||||||||||||||||||||||||||||||||||||||||||||||||||||||

You can definitely go and buy unpasteurized sauerkrauts at the store, and they are delicious! However, making kraut is extremely simple, easy, and affordable to do at home. I'm including the most basic recipe, but you can add many other things: beets, red cabbage, garlic, carrots, daikon, green onions...anything! Experiment!

MAKES ABOUT 1 QUART

1 medium head of cabbage

1½ tablespoons sea salt

EQUIPMENT:

½ gallon or quart-size mason jar or large slow cooker. (You need an opening large enough to put your hand in and tamp down the cabbage.)

Smaller jar filled with water or rocks. (This jar will sit on top of the cabbage and keep it submerged under the water.)

Good knife

Large mixing bowl

Dish towel

Rubber band

**Bonus:** Food processor and slicing attachment

1.  Make sure your mason jars and all surfaces are washed and thoroughly rinsed. You want to make sure the good bacteria have a fresh start to multiply.

2.  Take the outer leaves off of the cabbage and discard. Save one of the cleaner inner leaves, and set aside.

3.  Using a knife or a food processor, shred the cabbage.

4.  Place the cabbage in the mixing bowl and sprinkle with the sea salt. Mix thoroughly and allow to sit for 10 minutes.

5.  Begin squeezing and massaging cabbage. It takes about 5–10 minutes, so your forearms might get tired! You will squeeze until the cabbage is limp and you are able to squeeze out water.

6.  Place cabbage into the large mason jar and tamp down with your fist. Once all of the cabbage is inside, place the reserved whole cabbage leaf on top and tamp it down.

 *The* Nourished Belly Diet

7. Place the smaller jar filled with water or rocks on top of the cabbage. Use the jar to push the cabbage down. This jar stays in for the length of the ferment to keep the cabbage under water. Water should rise above the cabbage. If this doesn't happen, add 1 cup of water mixed with 1 tablespoon of salt.

8. Cover the jar with the dishcloth and seal with the rubber band so that nothing flies in, but air can still circulate.

9. Over the next day, check the cabbage every so often and make sure that it is completely submerged. The bacteria multiplies in an anaerobic environment, so we don't want the cabbage to be exposed to air.

10. Store the cabbage in a cool place that's out of the way. Kraut will ferment quicker in warmer temperatures. Be mindful if it's too hot because it has a tendency to become mushy and unappetizing.

11. Start tasting after 3 days. If there is a scummy layer that forms on top, simply discard it.

12. Small batches will ferment quicker than larger ones.

13. When you like the taste of the ferment, seal the jar with a lid and place in the refrigerator. Sauerkraut will last a few months, and if it starts to smell unappetizing, compost.

---

Experiment with different cabbages. Savoy and Napa make great krauts.

---

# Ghee

||||||||||||||||||||||||||||||||||||||||||||||||||||||||||||||||||||||||||||||||||||||||||||||||||||||||||||||||||||||

Since it is so simple and relatively quick to make, I don't make large batches of ghee at once. I use it pretty frequently, so I keep it in my pantry, which keeps it soft and easy to scoop out. After 3 or 4 months, ghee loses its nutty aroma and starts to smell stale, so try to use it within 2 months. Relish using ghee: It has a long history and is extremely nourishing. It will add a beautiful flavor to your meals and add a foundation of clean, wholesome nutrition to your diet.

MAKES 2 CUPS

3 sticks unsalted organic butter

1 teaspoon thyme, rosemary, basil, or
garlic (optional)

1.  In a saucepan, heat the butter and herbs or garlic (if using) on low until it starts to simmer. A white foam will rise to the top, and it should start to bubble.

2.  When the foam starts to subside, tilt the saucepan to check the color of the solids at the bottom. Roughly 15 minutes after the start of simmering, they should turn golden brown and the ghee is done! Be careful not to burn the solids on the bottom, as this will affect the flavor.

3.  Strain and place in an opaque glass jar.

4.  Store the ghee in a cool, dark place.

# Homemade Yogurt

||||||||||||||||||||||||||||||||||||||||||||||||||||||||||||||||||||||||||||||||||||||||||||||||||||||||||||||

I've gone through periods when I've made my own yogurt. The thing I love about homemade yogurt is that it has a tang that store-bought brands don't have. This is due to the fact that the lactobacilli and other beneficial bacteria are eating the lactose (milk sugar) found in the milk. Most commercial yogurts are incubated for roughly 6 hours; those of us that make our own yogurt at home can incubate yogurt for 24 hours, and therefore, control for taste and amount of lactose leftover. The length of fermentation will ultimately depend on your own taste buds.

MAKES ROUGHLY 1 GALLON

1 gallon organic whole milk

½ cup leftover whole plain yogurt with live active cultures or yogurt starter kit

1.  Place the milk into a large stockpot. Simmer until milk reaches 180 degrees using a thermometer. This will kill off bacteria and give the starter a clean playground.

2.  Pour the milk into clean half-gallon mason jars and allow to cool.

3.  Split the yogurt between the jars and mix gently.

4.  Lid and place jars into the unheated oven or next to a warm, sunny window. An unheated oven usually stays around 100–110°F, which is ideal. If it is not warm enough, you can leave the light on.

5.  Taste periodically until the desired flavor is reached.

# Snacks

Snacks are awesome. They are another opportunity to get some great nourishment in, and they help to stave off cravings when you go too long without eating. I tend to think of snacks as mini meals in terms of the nutrition they give, and they *can* be mini meals.

Most importantly, for snacks, it helps if we are prepared. Sometimes I find myself out and about, and I stare longingly into my bag and just *wish* I had snacks in it. So I'll usually bring some nuts, and maybe a date bar with me, or an apple just so I have something when I feel the need.

Below are some delicious recipes to snack on at home, on the go, or at work if your place of employment has a fridge.

# Kale Chips

This recipe takes the mystery out of the $8 bag of kale chips at the store. You can make these at home, and it's pretty darn simple. Plus, it's a great substitute for something crunchy and salty that is way less healthy for you. Remember that kale is packed with nutrients—this could be a great way to get some nutrition into your picky eaters at home! I like to use the curly kind for this recipe.

**SERVES 2**

1 bunch kale

2 tablespoons extra virgin olive oil

sea salt, to taste

1.  Preheat oven to 350°F.

2.  Wash and dry kale, either using a salad spinner or paper towels.

3.  Tear kale apart into large chunks.

4.  Place kale into a large bowl.

5.  Add the olive oil and coat the kale using your hands.

6.  On a large baking sheet covered with parchment paper, place the kale pieces.

7.  Salt liberally and bake for roughly 15 minutes. Check periodically, because they can burn easily!

8.  Store in an airtight container. If kale becomes less crunchy, simply put it back into the oven for a quick crisp up.

# Sardine Nori Wraps

If you are like many of my clients, you are wrinkling your nose at the thought of sardines. Even my own mother hesitates to eat them. I made her this dish once, and she said to me in Taiwanese, "The first bite was the worst, and then I got used to it." I consider this to be one of her better reviews of my food! I've also made quite a few converts, however, partly because they do taste yummy and they are a powerhouse of nutrients. Conveniently canned and ready to eat, they provide lots of calcium (bones in!) and are a source of vitamins A and D. Sardines make a great addition to your pantry, especially for days when you need to whip up something nourishing in a hurry. I also love to just eat this sardine salad with crackers. Pretty much everything in this dish is optional; at its base are sardines and yogurt, which I sometimes eat on their own.

SERVES 2

2 tablespoons chopped red onion (optional)

2 tablespoons apple cider vinegar (optional)

1 can sardines in olive oil

2 tablespoons whole plain yogurt

¼ cup chopped green herb, such as cilantro, parsley, chives, or dill

¼ cup chopped pickles (optional)

¼ cup sauerkraut

1 nori sheet

½ medium carrot, grated

¼ avocado

handful of sprouts (optional)

1.  In a small bowl, soak the red onion in the apple cider vinegar and set aside. This step is optional.

2.  Open and drain the sardines and place them in a medium bowl.

3.  Mash the sardines with a fork and mix in the yogurt, herb, pickles, and sauerkraut.

4.  Mix in the red onion and the apple cider vinegar, if using.

5.  On a plate, lay down one nori sheet. You can hold the nori sheet over an open flame to crisp it up. (Hold it about 5 inches away from flame, flip it back and forth, and be careful not to burn it!)

6. On one end of the nori sheet, place the grated carrot and spread evenly.

7. Spread the sardine mixture over carrots.

8. Spread the avocado over the sardines.

9. Add sprouts to the top, if using.

10. Starting from one end, roll the wrap like a burrito until you have a nice, tight roll.

11. Eat immediately!

# Cilantro Mint Hummus

Hummus is a great way to get some protein and deliciousness into your day. The main ingredient is garbanzo beans, or chickpeas, which are a staple for vegetarians around the world. They are a great source of minerals and fiber.

I'm always tempted to buy hummus at the store when I'm looking for a snack but am constantly disappointed by all the additives listed on the back of the packages. It's simple enough to make yourself; that way, you'll know it's 100 percent nutritious. If you'd like to make a large batch and freeze some, then simply double this recipe.

MAKES ABOUT 3½ CUPS

1 cup dried or 2 cups canned garbanzo beans

1–2 quarts filtered water

1 cup loosely packed cilantro (with stems)

1–2 handfuls mint leaves

1 cup extra virgin olive oil

2 cloves garlic

3 heaping tablespoons tahini

¼ cup fresh lemon juice

zest from 1 lemon

¾ teaspoon sea salt, plus more to taste

pepper, to taste

1. Soak dried garbanzo beans overnight.

2. Throw out the soaking water and pour the chickpeas in a large saucepan, covering them with the filtered water. Boil for roughly 1 hour until soft.

3. Strain out chickpeas, but keep ¼ cup of the water and set aside.

4. Using either a large bowl (to use with an immersion blender), a food processor, or a blender, place in the garbanzo beans, cilantro, mint, olive oil, garlic, tahini, lemon juice, lemon zest, and salt. Blend everything until smooth.

5. Add in the reserved chickpea water or more olive oil until you get the desired consistency.

6. Add more salt and pepper until you get the desired taste. This will keep for about a week in the fridge.

||||||||||||||||||||||||||||||||||||||||||||||||||||||||||||||||||||||||||||||||||||||||||||||||||||||||||

**NOURISHING NOTE:** Experiment! You can incorporate cumin, turmeric, smoked paprika, curry powder, roasted red pepper, pumpkin seeds, and just about anything into hummus.

||||||||||||||||||||||||||||||||||||||||||||||||||||||||||||||||||||||||||||||||||||||||||||||||||||||||||

# Chicken Liver Paté

|||||||||||||||||||||||||||||||||||||||||||||||||||||||||||||||||||||||||||||||||||||||||||||||||||||||||||||||||

Livers are one of the most nutrient-dense foods that you can eat. Their nutrient profile is incredible: vitamins A, D, E, K, and B12, folic acid, and minerals such as copper and iron. So when you consume the livers of healthy animals, you are also getting a dose of amazing vitamins! (Liver is not recommended for those with gout.) Making paté is a wonderful way to eat liver. Spread it on sandwiches or crackers, or dip it with cut veggies. Feel free to experiment with the recipe by adding cooked mushrooms, turmeric, or cloves.

MAKES ROUGHLY 3 CUPS

4 tablespoons cold butter, cubed

1 large yellow onion, sliced

1 pint organic chicken livers

2 teaspoons chopped fresh thyme (optional)

2 teaspoons chopped fresh sage (optional)

2 teaspoons chopped fresh rosemary (optional)

2–3 teaspoons miso OR ½ tablespoon sea salt

salt and pepper, to taste

1. In a medium sauté pan, melt 1 tablespoon of the butter.

2. Add the onion and sauté until translucent.

3. Add the livers and herbs, if using.

4. Sauté the livers until the insides are still slightly pink. Allow liver/onion mixture to cool.

5. Transfer liver, onions, and herbs, if using, into a mixing bowl.

6. Add miso or salt, and the rest of the cubed butter.

7. Use an immersion blender and blend.

8. Add salt and pepper, to taste. Blend.

9. Jar and allow mixture to cool; place in fridge for a firmer texture before enjoying!

# Seasonal Fruit Parfait

|||||||||||||||||||||||||||||||||||||||||||||||||||||||||||||||||||||||||||||||||||||||||||||||||||||||

Fruits are such an amazing seasonal treat. There are fruits in every season that I get excited about. Whether they be the watermelon and peaches in the summer or the persimmons in the fall, they are all so incredibly delicious. They really are nature's candy. I love making homemade fruit parfaits because store-bought ones usually include flavored yogurt. Plus, pairing fruit with yogurt follows the idea of eating carbs with fat. Boost the nutrition by adding belly boosters!

MAKES 1 SERVING

1 cup seasonal fruit, such as berries, peaches, or soft persimmons

1 cup whole plain yogurt

¼ cup cashews, almonds, or pecans

1.  Using a tall container or glass, arrange the yogurt and fruit in multiple layers.

2.  Add the nuts as a garnish.

3.  Enjoy immediately, or transfer to a mason jar for a snack later on!

# Breakfast

I love breakfast. It's so important! It helps set up your metabolism for the rest of the day and ensures that you aren't dropping in energy around 3 or 4 p.m., reaching for that next cup of coffee. One gem that I love to tell my clients is to think about having dinner for breakfast! There's no rule book that says breakfast must only be eggs and bacon.

According to traditional Chinese medicine, each organ has a peak function time. The stomach's time is from 7 to 9 a.m., when digestion is very strong. So following this organ clock, eating between 7 and 9 a.m. is ideal! Also, take into consideration that it's good to eat within 45 minutes to an hour of waking.

# Sweet Millet Cereal

Millet is a nutty-tasting grain that is a wonderful addition to the breakfast porridge rotation. It's one of the grains with a higher protein content compared to corn and rice, and is also a good source of minerals and B vitamins. Note: Those with hypothyroid shouldn't consume millet on a regular basis since it has a substance that can interfere with thyroid function.

MAKES 5 CUPS

1 cup millet

4 cups water

2 cups coconut milk

½ cup raisins

2 eggs

2 tablespoons chia seeds

1 tablespoon maple syrup

$\frac{1}{16}$ teaspoon sea salt

1. Place the millet in medium saucepan with the water and coconut milk.

2. Add the raisins. Simmer with a lid on for 20–25 minutes.

3. Stir in the eggs, chia seeds, maple syrup, and salt.

4. Let sit, covered, for 5–10 minutes.

5. Experiment with different toppings and enjoy!

# Power Oatmeal

A great replacement for packaged cereals, oatmeal is part of a healthy diet. Oats are one of the few foods that have been studied extensively, and they have been shown to lower cholesterol. It's something that you can batch cook and keep in your fridge for use throughout the week.

This recipe also includes the step of soaking your oats the night before. Most grains include phytic acid, which will bind to many minerals. When we soak grains with some apple cider vinegar, this helps to activate the enzyme phytase, which breaks down the phytic acid. You will not completely reduce all the phytic acid, but this is a nice habit to get into. Don't stress if you forget this step!

SERVES 2

1 cup rolled or steel cut oats

½ cup coconut milk

1¼ cups filtered water, as needed

handful of raisins

handful of coconut flakes

1 medium egg (optional)

½ cup seasonal fruit

handful of sunflower seeds or other nuts

1 teaspoon ground flaxseeds

1. The night before, soak oats in 1 cup of water and a splash of apple cider vinegar.

2. The next morning, spoon out desired amount, and refrigerate the rest.

3. Place the oats in a small saucepan with the coconut milk and ¼ cup of water.

4. Add raisins and coconut flakes and cook for approximately 5 minutes.

5. The mixture should be slightly soupy, not too firm. If too firm, add a tiny bit more coconut milk or water.

6. Crack the egg into mixture, if using, and stir until incorporated, but do not overcook. Whites should not be translucent. Remove pan from heat.

7. Add fruit, sunflower seeds, flaxseeds, and other desired toppings.

# Savory Oatmeal

||||||||||||||||||||||||||||||||||||||||||||||||||||||||||||||||||||||||||||||||||||||||||||||||||||

Oats don't always have to be sweet! They are great savory as well and are a quick, delicious, warming meal. This recipe includes the belly boosters flax and kelp. These are both optional, but remember, you are trying to make every meal as nutrient-filled as possible, and these two are great additions. Flax for healthy fatty acids, and kelp for a nice dose of iodine and minerals! If you don't have time to soak the oats, use dried oats and increase the water to 1 cup.

SERVES 1

½ cup soaked oats

½ cup filtered water

1 medium egg

1 teaspoon ground flaxseeds

⅛ teaspoon toasted sesame oil

¹⁄₁₆ teaspoon sea salt

sprinkle of kelp (optional)

1. Place the soaked oats in a saucepan with the filtered water.

2. Bring to a boil on medium heat, and then simmer on low.

3. Cook for 5 minutes, stirring occasionally.

4. Turn off heat, crack egg into oats, and stir until the egg is incorporated.

5. Add the flaxseeds, sesame oil, sea salt, and kelp, if using.

6. Taste and adjust accordingly. Enjoy!

# Power Smoothie

||||||||||||||||||||||||||||||||||||||||||||||||||||||||||||||||||||||||||||||||||||||||||||||||||

Smoothies are ideal for the busy person, especially on days when you are on the run. Remember variety! You can put just about anything in smoothies and they usually come out pretty tasty. They also hide strong flavors like algae and fish oils well.

SERVES 2

1 banana

1 cup seasonal fruit, such as berries, peaches, or pears

½ cooked sweet potato with skin on (optional)

½ cup coconut milk

½ cup plain whole yogurt

1 tablespoon freshly ground flaxseeds

1 teaspoon chia seeds

1 tablespoon nut butter of choice

dash of kelp powder

dash of spirulina or chlorella

filtered water

1. Put all ingredients into a blender and blend. Add in water until you get the desired consistency. You can even make it the night before, but be warned that the ground flaxseeds and chia will make it more like a gel than a smoothie. You might need to eat it with a spoon!

# Coconut Banana Squash Pancakes

||||||||||||||||||||||||||||||||||||||||||||||||||||||||||||||||||||||||||||||||||||||||||||||||||||||||||||||

Pancakes are an American brunch staple. I'm excited to share this recipe for coconut flour pancakes, which also make great on-the-go snacks. Spread some almond butter on them and they work as a post-workout snack. They are denser than normal pancakes, so don't expect the same fluffiness, but they are wonderful in their own way. My favorite way to eat them is dipped in yogurt.

SERVES 2

1 ripe banana

2 eggs

⅛ teaspoon vanilla

2 heaping tablespoons cooked squash, canned pumpkin, or sweet potato

3 tablespoons coconut flour

⅛ teaspoon ground cinnamon

handful of coconut shreds

⅛ teaspoon salt

⅛ teaspoon baking powder

3 tablespoons coconut oil or butter

1. Heat a large sauté pan on the stove while you mash the banana, eggs, vanilla, and squash in a medium bowl with an immersion blender or mixer.

2. Add the coconut flour, cinnamon, coconut shreds, salt, and baking powder. Mix thoroughly with a spatula.

3. Turn heat to low, and place 1 tablespoon of coconut oil or butter per batch in the sauté pan.

4. Cook for roughly 2 minutes on low on each side. Be careful flipping!

5. Enjoy with fruit, maple syrup, nut butter, yogurt, or any topping you wish!

# Quinoa Bites

||||||||||||||||||||||||||||||||||||||||||||||||||||||||||||||||||||||||||||||||||||||||||||||||||||||

My client Tonya introduced me to these (shout out to Tonya!). She was inspired through Pinterest, and once she started making them, she discovered they are a game changer.

Cook these ahead of time, store them in the fridge (freeze, too, for later), or grab them on the go. They're a quick way to get in a whole foods breakfast, and kids love them. They are also a clever way to use leftover veggies, because you can really put anything in them. Below is a combination that I have found particularly crowd pleasing, and they are just so *cute*.

MAKES 12 BITES

2–3 strips bacon

4 eggs

1 teaspoon sea salt

2 cups sliced zucchini

2 cup sliced mushrooms (any kind)

2 cups cooked quinoa

3 cloves garlic

1 small yellow onion, diced

1 tablespoon coconut oil

dash of black pepper

1. Warm a sauté pan over medium heat.

2. Place the bacon slices in the pan and cook for 2–3 minutes on each side or until crispy. Watch so they don't burn!

3. Once the bacon is crispy, remove and set aside on a plate.

4. Preheat oven to 375°F.

5. Crack eggs on countertop and place them into bowl.

6. Mix well with a fork, and add salt.

7. Add the sliced zucchini, mushrooms, quinoa, garlic, and onion to egg mixture.

8. Slice the bacon into smaller pieces. Add it to the egg mixture and mix well.

9. Add in dash of pepper and mix.

10. Use the coconut oil to grease the sides of a standard 12-cup muffin tin.

11. For extra-easy removal, cut strips of parchment paper and line the middle of each muffin cup.

12. Divide mixture evenly into the cups; feel free to fill them generously since the mixture will cook down.

13. Bake for 30 minutes, then remove and let cool slightly.

14. Enjoy! If storing, allow to cool completely before refrigerating or freezing.

# Hearty Rice Porridge (Congee)

||||||||||||||||||||||||||||||||||||||||||||||||||||||||||||||||||||||||||||||||||||||||||||||||||||||||

Congee is a complete comfort food that can be eaten at any time of day. My family used to eat this on Sunday mornings with side dishes of dried pork, pickled vegetables, and fish. I usually make a big pot from leftover rice, and either invite friends over for a traditional Taiwanese brunch or keep the rest in the fridge to pull out for a warming meal.

Congee is great for those who are sick and need something easily digestible to get them back on their feet. Congee originated from the Chinese culture. In Taiwan, the month after a mother gives birth is called *zuo yue zi*, or the sitting month. During this time, she must follow some interesting rules: she can't bathe and must be wrapped up all the time! Rice porridge is a star food during this important time for the mother to regain her energy and strength.

SERVES 3–4

2 cups day-old rice

1 quart bone broth or vegetable broth

2 cups water (if needed)

1. On the stovetop, combine the rice and broth in a large saucepan, and bring to a simmer.

2. Stir every 10 minutes or so, adding water as needed to keep the congee from sticking to the bottom of the pot.

3. Cook until you are happy with the consistency, usually around an hour.

**NOURISHING NOTE:**

CONGEE ADDITIONS:

- Dried shiitake mushrooms: Soak these for an hour or so in filtered water. When soft, slice and add both the soaking water and the mushrooms to the congee.

- Kombu or wakame: Kombu is a heartier seaweed that can be added in the beginning; wakame can be added at the end.

- Pulled chicken or pork: Anytime you have leftover meat, thinly slicing or pulling into chunks make a great addition to the congee.

YUMMY COMBINATIONS:

- With a fried egg and sardines
- With cooked kale and pulled pork
- With kimchee and salmon

# Huevos Pericos

One of my closest girlfriends, Vanessa, is Colombian. She introduced me to this dish a few years ago when we traveled to Colombia, frolicked around the markets, and ate our way through the country. I've seen this recipe made with scallions and green onions, but this is how I learned it from Vanessa, who learned it from her mother. It's a surprisingly simple dish with few ingredients, but it's great over rice or with tortillas as well. It's my go-to when I have friends over for brunch because it's so simple, and I always receive compliments.

**SERVES 2**

1 large pat butter

1 medium yellow onion, chopped

4 eggs

1 large tomato, chopped

salt and pepper, to taste

tortillas or greens, to serve

1. Heat a medium sauté pan for a minute or so on the stovetop before putting in butter.

2. Add the chopped onion and stir until it is translucent, roughly 3–4 minutes.

3. While onion is cooking, crack the eggs into a small mixing bowl. Whip them with a fork until completely mixed.

4. Add chopped tomatoes to the onion and let cook for roughly 2 minutes, stirring occasionally.

5. Add in eggs, and stir frequently, letting the eggs become more of a mixed scramble.

6. Cook to the desired doneness.

7. Add salt and pepper.

8. Enjoy on tortillas or on top of greens!

*The* Nourished Belly Diet

# Salads and Sauces

Salad dressings and sauces used to perplex me. *What is in here that makes it so good?* Since everything was always blended together, it seemed like such an enigma that I didn't know how to crack. Now, like all things that take some experimentation and reading up on, they really aren't all that hard. Sauces are great because they can be dips, or you can mix a little more olive oil, water, or yogurt in them, and they become salad dressings! I've definitely made some mistakes in combinations I *thought* would be good, but I've learned my lesson. Here are some simple combinations I use in my kitchen.

# Super-Basic Vinaigrette

The most basic thing you could place on your salad is oil and vinegar. The good news is that there are lots of different vinegars out there to try, and different oils too, but my staple is extra virgin olive oil. As for the acidic portion, try red wine vinegar, apple cider vinegar, a high-quality balsamic vinegar (it should be thick), sherry vinegar, lemon juice, umeboshi plum vinegar, or rice wine vinegar.

YIELD DEPENDS ON YOU!

1 part vinegar

3 parts extra virgin olive oil

pinch of salt and pepper

1.  Think about how much salad dressing you need; if it's just for a small dinner party, a tablespoon of vinegar is enough. For larger parties, perhaps use a quarter cup.

2.  Place the vinegar in a bowl and add a pinch of salt. Taste it, the salt should take some of the acidity away.

3.  Sprinkle in some black pepper.

4.  Add olive oil and whisk together. Serve immediately!

# Seasonal Pumpkin Seed Pesto

Packed with nutrients, traditional pesto with basil and pine nuts consists of light, summery flavors. Basil is great to use during its summer peak but I like to change the recipe based on the season. Cilantro is my herb of choice in winter; however, feel free to use any leafy green, including spinach, parsley, and blanched nettles. You can also substitute any fatty nut or seed: Pumpkin seeds, sunflower seeds, macadamia nuts, and walnuts are all delicious choices. This recipes does not include Parmesan, which you of course can add, but without it this is dairy free, and plus, I don't like freezing cheese!

MAKES ROUGHLY 2 CUPS

2 cups leafy green or herb

¾ cup extra virgin olive oil

⅔ cup pumpkin seeds or other nuts or seeds of your choice

2–3 cloves garlic

½ teaspoon sea salt

juice of one lemon

1. Combine all of the ingredients in a food processor or bowl with an immersion blender.

2. Taste, and add more salt or lemon juice if necessary.

3. Store in an airtight container for up to a week in the fridge, or freeze in ice cube trays for later use.

# Tahini Miso Dressing

Tahini is delicious. It's made from toasted, ground hulled sesame seeds, which are belly boosters (see page 52) and powerhouses of healthy fats, high protein, and minerals. Sesame seeds alone are great to add to salads and salad dressings, and the tahini itself has a beautiful flavor that is great in its own dressing. You might recognize it as one of the main ingredients in hummus.

This dressing also includes the belly booster miso, which, along with healthy probiotics, is a more absorbable form of soy. Use this dressing as a dipping sauce for veggies, or on your favorite salad.

SERVES 6

2 tablespoons unsalted tahini

1 tablespoon white miso

⅛ teaspoon sesame oil

½ tablespoon fresh lemon juice

1 teaspoon honey

3 tablespoons filtered water

1. Place all ingredients into a small bowl and mix until smooth.

# Honey Miso Dressing

SERVES 6

3 tablespoons brown or white organic miso

2 tablespoons apple cider vinegar

1 teaspoon honey

¼ cup extra virgin olive oil

¼ cup toasted sesame oil

1 teaspoon wheat-free tamari

1. Pour miso, vinegar, and honey together in a bowl and mix until smooth.

2. Add olive oil, sesame oil, and tamari. Taste. If too vinegary, add more oil. If too salty, add more honey. If too oily, add more miso! Experiment!

# Cashew Garlic Cream

||||||||||||||||||||||||||||||||||||||||||||||||||||||||||||||||||||||||||||||||||||||||||||||||||||||||

This is a gold mine—really. It goes well on top of *everything*. It pairs particularly well with polenta, but it's also great on greens, mixed in with salad. I just can't get enough of it.

MAKES 1½ CUPS (ROUGHLY 12 SERVINGS)

| | |
|---|---|
| 1 cup soaked cashews | 2 teaspoons fresh lemon juice |
| ½ cup filtered water | zest from 1 lemon |
| 1 large clove garlic | salt, to taste (roughly ½ teaspoon) |

1. Drain the cashews and place them into a blender.

2. Add the water, garlic, lemon juice, and zest.

3. Blend on high until smooth.

4. Taste, and add salt as desired.

5. Feel free to add more garlic, lemon juice, or water until the cream reaches the desired taste and consistency.

# Mango Cilantro Salad

||||||||||||||||||||||||||||||||||||||||||||||||||||||||||||||||||||||||||||||||||||||||||||||||||||

This is a Mama Chang recipe. My mother excels at throwing dinner parties, and one of the main activities that she and the other Taiwanese moms do is swap recipes. I'm not sure where she got this party favorite from, but it's excellent.

SERVES 4–6

2 large mangos (1 unripe and 1 slightly ripe), cubed

2 teaspoons sea salt

1 tablespoon toasted sesame oil

2 teaspoons fresh lemon juice and zest from 1 lemon

½ cup roughly chopped cilantro

1 sliced avocado (optional)

1 cup cooked freshwater shrimp (optional)

1. Place the mango cubes into a large bowl and sprinkle with the sea salt.

2. Mix the mangoes pieces until they are evenly coated. Let sit for 10 minutes, and drain.

3. Add the sesame oil, lemon juice, and lemon zest. Add more oil, to taste, if necessary.

4. Finally, mix in the chopped cilantro until evenly dispersed. You can garnish with a few sprigs for presentation!

5. Add the avocado and shrimp for a heartier meal.

# Quinoa, Mint, and Red Onion Salad

One of my favorite things about quinoa is that it works great cold in a salad with whatever you have in your fridge. The base here is the quinoa, apple cider vinegar, and olive oil, and the rest can be whatever you want. Just use color as your guide and you can't go wrong. The flavors below work great together, so start there. This recipe is best used with leftover, refrigerated quinoa.

SERVES 4–6

½ diced red onion

¼ cup apple cider vinegar

2 cups cooked quinoa

4 sprigs finely minced mint

1 medium carrot, grated

handful of chopped nuts (any kind)

¼ cup raisins or currants

⅛ teaspoon salt

¼ cup crumbled feta cheese (optional)

1 tablespoon extra virgin olive oil

black pepper, to taste

1.  Soak the red onion in the apple cider vinegar for about 10–15 minutes or until the onion is translucent.

2.  Combine the quinoa and mint in a large bowl.

3.  Add the carrot, nuts, raisins or currants, salt, and feta, if using.

4.  Add the red onion and 2–3 tablespoons of the apple cider vinegar.

5.  Mix thoroughly and add olive oil. Taste. Add in more vinegar, salt, and pepper as desired.

# Massaged Chicken and Kale Salad with Honey Miso Dressing

||||||||||||||||||||||||||||||||||||||||||||||||||||||||||||||||||||||||||||||||||||||||||||||||||||||||||||||||||

This is the recipe that I use most often when I do a cooking demo or show clients how to make something quick. It's a great way to eat kale without having to cook it, although it's debatable whether it saves more time. In any case, it's a nice way to enjoy kale in a salad, and because you massage the kale, it's more digestible than just eating it raw. Any type of kale will do; I like lacinato. For the fruit chunks, apple, pear, persimmon, or grapes work well.

**SERVES 2**

1 sliced pear or apple

1 bunch kale

Honey Miso Dressing (page 124)

¼ cup chopped walnuts

1 cup pulled chicken

salt and pepper, to taste

1 pear, apple, or other seasonal fruit, sliced

1. Place the pear or apple in a bowl of lightly salted water to prevent browning. Set aside.

2. Wash the kale and remove the stems by squeezing the stem and pulling down on the leaf. Roll leaves together like a burrito and thinly slice across to make small, thin ribbons. Place in a large bowl, and sprinkle with salt and pepper.

3. With clean hands, massage the kale, squeezing and mixing until it turns a bright green.

4. In a small bowl, thoroughly mix the walnuts and pulled chicken with 1 tablespoon of Honey Miso Dressing. Taste, and add more dressing if necessary.

5. Plate each serving with a handful of kale. Add the chicken and walnuts. Sprinkle with fruit chunks.

6. Enjoy!

# Colorful Cabbage Salad

Whenever I need something quick and easy to bring to a potluck, I love to make a colorful cabbage salad that's full of phytonutrients. Most people are surprised by how good raw cabbage can be.

SERVES 6–8

2 apples, sliced into chunks

½ head green cabbage, cored and cut into bite-size slivers

½ head purple cabbage, cored and cut into bite-size slivers

2 medium carrots, grated

½ teaspoon salt

1½ tablespoons rice wine vinegar

1½ tablespoons extra virgin olive oil

2 handfuls of sunflower seeds

2 handfuls of raisins

1. Place the apples in a bowl of slightly salted water to prevent browning. Set aside.

2. Place the green and purple cabbage into a large bowl.

3. Add the carrots.

4. Drain the apples and mix them in.

5. Sprinkle with the salt and mix.

6. Add the vinegar, olive oil, sunflower seeds, and raisins.

7. Taste. Add more of any ingredient as desired.

8. Serve!

# Tomato Corn Basil Salad

||||||||||||||||||||||||||||||||||||||||||||||||||||||||||||||||||||||||||||||||||||||||||||||||||||||||

Showcase summer's bounty with this quick salad, which doesn't take a whole lot of seasoning when you buy the ingredients at their peak. There are few ingredients, and it's definitely a crowd-pleaser. You could add mozzarella for a classic buffalo salad; peppers, peaches, and watermelon also make nice additions.

**SERVES 2**

kernels from 1 cob of corn

2 ripe tomatoes, roughly chopped

sea salt and pepper, to taste

about 8 julienned basil leaves

2 teaspoons high-quality balsamic vinegar

1 tablespoon extra virgin olive oil

1. Place corn kernels in a large bowl. (You can save the corn cob for veggie broth!)

2. Place the tomatoes in, being careful not to lose the juice!

3. Sprinkle with the sea salt and pepper. (You could add the basil here and be done if you like!)

4. Add the balsamic and olive oil. Lightly mix.

5. Garnish with basil and serve!

# Carrot Beet Salad

I love the color that this salad adds to the plate—it fits perfectly in the Nourished Bowl. This is a perfect dish to bring to a potluck or dinner party. It's always a huge hit! The carrots and beets add sweetness and, if you are doing dairy, the feta adds a nice, salty creaminess. Plus, every ingredient in this salad is full of nutrients that, with some healthy fats, help us to detox and clear out free radicals. During the summer months, this salad is great mixed with pesto, or if you have leftovers, you can combine with cooked quinoa for a quick salad.

**SERVES 4**

2 medium beets, grated

4 medium carrots, grated

½ cup chopped green herb, such as cilantro, mint, or parsley

salt and pepper, to taste

1 tablespoon extra virgin olive oil

2 teaspoons apple cider, balsamic, or rice vinegar

½ cup feta (optional)

2 tablespoons hemp seeds

1.  Place the beets and carrots in a large bowl.

2.  Add the green herbs, and sprinkle with salt and pepper, then add the olive oil and vinegar.

3.  Toss well and add feta, if desired.

4.  Sprinkle with hemp seeds.

5.  Enjoy with a nice side of polenta, greens, and piece of chicken or steak!

# Veggie Sides

When I read my clients' diet journals, the largest, most prominent piece missing is the inclusion of daily vegetables. Salad appears often, but vegetables have so much more to offer than just salad! Plus, I am an advocate of eating cooked, warm foods, especially in the cooler months, and we benefit from eating cooked vegetables.

When you really start to experiment with eating vegetables and cutting out processed foods, your taste buds start to realize how sweet an ear of corn and a stem of broccoli can be, not to mention the myriad of health benefits, from fiber to phytonutrients, you get when you eat a diet full of veggies.

Let's start experimenting! Below are the recipes I use most often. What's great about them is that they are simple and quick to make. I often tell clients to buy something they've never seen or heard of before and to challenge themselves to learn how to make it. So challenge yourself!

# Bok Choy, Mushrooms, and Garlic

Bok choy is a great side dish because it cooks so darn fast. If you really need to whip something up in a hurry, this is it.

SERVES 2–3

1 large pat butter or 1 tablespoon ghee or cooking oil

½ cup sliced mushrooms (any kind)

2 tablespoons water or broth

3 bunches bok choy, chopped in ¼-inch slices

2 cloves garlic, minced

2 teaspoons soy sauce or wheat-free tamari

1. In a large sauté pan over medium heat, melt the butter, ghee, or cooking oil, and throw in the mushrooms.

2. Add the 2 tablespoons of water or broth and stir.

3. When the mushrooms start to wilt, add the bok choy and garlic.

4. Add the soy sauce or tamari and more water, if necessary.

5. Cook for approximately 4 minutes until wilted and dark green, then remove from heat and enjoy.

# Bacon and Collards

IIIIIIIIIIIIIIIIIIIIIIIIIIIIIIIIIIIIIIIIIIIIIIIIIIIIIIIIIIIIIIIIIIIIIIIIIIIIIIIIIIIIIIIIIIIII

Having lived for six years in North Carolina, I discovered that bacon and collards are staples in the South. Plus, bacon is full of umami, the natural flavor enhancer. You can substitute the collard greens in this classic recipe with pretty much any leafy green.

SERVES 2–3

3 slices pastured, nitrate-free bacon

1 bunch collard greens, sliced or roughly chopped

2 cloves garlic, minced

splash of water or broth

1. Warm a medium sauté pan over medium heat.

2. Place bacon slices in pan and cook for 2–3 minutes on each side or until crispy. Watch so they don't burn!

3. Once bacon is crispy, remove and set aside on a plate.

4. In the same pan with the bacon fat (yes!), add in the sliced greens and minced garlic.

5. Sauté for roughly 3–4 minutes, add the water or broth, and cover for a minute or two.

6. Place greens on a plate, crumble bacon on top, and serve.

# Summertime Gazpacho

||||||||||||||||||||||||||||||||||||||||||||||||||||||||||||||||||||||||||||||||||||||||||||||||

Gazpacho originates from the southern region of Spain, and I first learned in high school Spanish class, when my first thought was, "Cold soup?" However, the first time someone made it for me from fresh ingredients, I was forever changed. It's a perfect hot, sunny day dish, and when you make it with ingredients available at the peak of the summer season, you can't go wrong.

SERVES 3–4

1½ pounds (roughly 5 medium) ripe tomatoes, chopped

1 medium yellow or red bell pepper, roughly chopped

1 medium cucumber, roughly chopped

2 cloves garlic

1 teaspoon balsamic vinegar

¾ teaspoon salt

2 tablespoons extra virgin olive oil, plus more to garnish (optional)

black pepper, to taste

toasted pumpkin seeds, to garnish (optional)

avocado, to garnish (optional)

chopped chives, to garnish (optional)

1. Combine all of the ingredients except the pumpkin seeds, avocado, and chives in a food processor or blender and pulse until finely chopped.

2. Pour into a bowl.

3. Cover and chill for a few hours before serving. Garnish as desired.

# Eggplant and Peppers
# with Cashew Garlic Cream

||||||||||||||||||||||||||||||||||||||||||||||||||||||||||||||||||||||||||||||||||||||||||

Some people are dead set against eggplant. It's the texture, they say. For me, that is exactly why I love eggplant: the texture! It's a wonderful source of fiber and phytonutrients. Plus, it takes on other flavors really well and is a hearty addition to a meal. This dish is perfectly fine on its own with some sea salt and black pepper, with pesto, or the way I have it here, with Garlic Cashew Cream. Make a bunch so that you can eat it throughout the week.

**SERVES 4**

1 tablespoon coconut oil

1 small yellow onion, sliced

1 red bell pepper, sliced

1 green bell pepper, sliced

2 long purple eggplants, sliced thinly

splash of filtered water or broth

½ cup Cashew Garlic Cream (page 125)

salt and pepper

1. Heat the coconut oil in a large sauté pan on low to medium heat.

2. Cook the onion on low until they are semi-translucent, stirring frequently.

3. Add the bell peppers and the eggplant with the filtered water or broth. Stir and cover.

4. Let the veggies cook for roughly 10 minutes or until the eggplant has changed into an opaque color and you can run a fork through easily.

5. Remove from heat.

6. Mix in the Cashew Garlic Cream.

7. Add salt and pepper.

8. Plate and serve.

# Roasted Brussels Sprouts and Bacon

I used to dislike brussels sprouts for no more reason than in children's books, the main characters always seemed to wrinkle their noses at them. As an adult, I saw that brussels sprouts are really mini cabbages! How cool. They also have the same liver detox benefits that cabbage does. Plus, they have a sweetness to them that is delicious, and they are great roasted. I also like to thinly slice them and do a quick sauté.

SERVES 3–4

15–20 brussels sprouts, sliced in half

6 cloves garlic with the skin on

4 slices of pastured bacon

sea salt and pepper, to taste

1. Preheat the oven to 375°F.

2. Place brussels sprouts on a baking sheet.

3. Scatter the garlic cloves on the same baking sheet.

4. Place the bacon slices on top of the vegetables.

5. Roast in the oven for 35–45 minutes, checking to make sure the bacon isn't burning and checking the brussels sprouts for doneness by sticking a fork in them.

6. When a fork slides easily through the brussels sprouts, remove tray from oven and place in large serving dish.

7. Leave bacon as is, cut into smaller pieces, or crumble on top.

8. Sprinkle with salt and pepper, and enjoy!

# Garlic Cauliflower Mash

||||||||||||||||||||||||||||||||||||||||||||||||||||||||||||||||||||||||||||||||||||||||||||||||||||||

Cauliflower and garlic are both excellent for liver detoxification. Cauliflower is part of the brassica or crucifer family, as are brussels sprouts, broccoli, and cabbage. These veggies are great for liver health, as is garlic! This is an excellent substitute for mashed potatoes. Great for those sensitive to nightshades, which include tomatoes, eggplant, pepper, and potatoes.

SERVES ABOUT 6

1 large (about 1 pound) cauliflower, cut into florets

5 cloves garlic, peeled

2 teaspoons butter or coconut oil

¼ teaspoon ground cumin

salt and pepper, to taste

1.  Fill a large saucepan with roughly an inch of water. Add the cauliflower and garlic, then cover the pan with a lid and steam for 10 minutes, until you can pierce the cauliflower with a fork.

2.  Put cauliflower, garlic, cumin, and butter or oil into a blender or food processor, or use a hand blender and whip until smooth.

3.  Add salt and pepper.

4.  Serve like mashed potatoes.

# Coconut Kale

This was my most-used recipe when I first started eating kale; it's a great way to add a bit of sweetness when you are first learning to cook kale, and the coconut flavor is lovely. Plus, the healthy fats from the coconut are necessary to help you fully absorb the nutrients from the kale, so this is a great pairing.

SERVES 2–3

1 heaping teaspoon coconut oil

1 bunch any type kale, roughly chopped

1 tablespoon coconut shreds

¼ cup coconut milk

1 clove garlic, minced

1 teaspoon soy sauce

1. In a large sauté pan, heat a spoonful of coconut oil over medium heat.

2. Add the chopped kale, stirring to make sure each leaf is covered with the oil.

3. Add the coconut shreds and coconut milk, then cover for about 45 seconds.

4. Uncover and add the minced garlic, stirring continuously until the kale leaves are wilted and have turned a nice, dark green.

5. Add the soy sauce and serve!

# Aloo Gobi

||||||||||||||||||||||||||||||||||||||||||||||||||||||||||||||||||||||||||||||||||||||||||||||||||||

Indian dishes are lovely because of the colorful spice blends. It's easy to make this dish flavorful, and it just feels oh so comforting! Aloo Gobi is an Indian dish that literally means cauliflower and potatoes. This is a hearty dish as is; sometimes I add a few chicken drums for flavor and healthy fats.

SERVES 4

2 tablespoons coconut oil

1 large yellow onion, chopped

1 teaspoon cumin seeds

2 teaspoon turmeric

2 teaspoon garam masala

1 (12-ounce) BPA-free can or glass jar (about 2 large) tomatoes

1 tablespoon fresh ginger, minced

3 cloves garlic, minced

½ large cauliflower, chopped into small florets

3 large potatoes, skin on, chopped in cubes

1 teaspoon sea salt

3 handfuls of roughly chopped cilantro, plus more to garnish

1.  On the stovetop, heat a large sauté pan over medium heat, and when warm, add the coconut oil.

2.  Add the onion and cumin seeds. Stir periodically until the onion is translucent.

3.  Add the turmeric and garam masala. Give a quick stir.

4.  Add the tomatoes, ginger, and garlic. Stir.

5.  Add the cauliflower and potatoes. Cover and simmer for 20 minutes, periodically checking and stirring. Add a little water if anything starts to stick to the bottom.

6.  Simmer until cauliflower and potatoes are soft enough that a fork can stick through easily.

7.  Add salt and taste, adding more if necessary.

8.  Mix in a few handfuls of fresh cilantro, and garnish the top before serving.

9.  Serve with brown rice or quinoa.

 *The* Nourished Belly Diet

# Basic Roasted Winter Squash

||||||||||||||||||||||||||||||||||||||||||||||||||||||||||||||||||||||||||||||||||||||||||||||||||||||||||||||||||

One of the reasons why I love fall is that winter squash comes into season. Talk about natural, sweet goodness. This is a beautiful way to curb a sweet tooth and add sweetness into any dish. This recipe is a perfect complement to the Slow Cooked Pork Ribs (page 165) and the Homestyle Ground Beef (page 152). Plus, the leftover squash can be used for the Coconut Banana Squash Pancakes (page 115).

These go in the oven naked so you could use them with many recipes, but you could definitely add butter and cinnamon before putting them in. Try this recipe using kabocha, butternut, acorn, or delicata squash. Save the seeds and roast them separately, if you like.

SERVES 3–4

1 winter squash, halved

melted butter, to serve

1. Preheat the oven to 375°F.

2. On a baking sheet covered with parchment paper, place the squash halves, open side down.

3. Roast in the oven for 45 minutes or until a fork slides easily through.

4. Serve immediately with melted butter, or let cool, scoop out, and store in jars for later meals!

||||||||||||||||||||||||||||||||||||||||||||||||||||||||||||||||||||||||||||||||||||||||||||||||||||||||||||||||||

**NOURISHING NOTE:** Winter squash has great health benefits, including anti-inflammatory, antioxidant, and insulin-regulating properties. Look for ones with firm rinds, as softness can signal spoilage. Remember to eat these vegetables with a healthy fat to ensure maximum nutrient absorption! I recommend organic, grass-fed butter and coconut oil.

||||||||||||||||||||||||||||||||||||||||||||||||||||||||||||||||||||||||||||||||||||||||||||||||||||||||||||||||||

# Basic Roasted Sweet Potato

||||||||||||||||||||||||||||||||||||||||||||||||||||||||||||||||||||||||||||||||||||||||||||||||||||||||

Sweet potatoes are versatile and are great for diabetics since they have plenty of fiber to slow the release of blood sugar. They are extremely nutritious; make sure you have a bit of fat when you eat them so that all the nutrients can be easily absorbed. I prefer to roast them because it brings out the sweetness.

The orange ones are often called yams but are technically sweet potatoes. These are often more watery and do not hold up as well in stews. They also do not take as long to roast. The purple ones are my favorites for stews and home fries.

This recipe will make enough to enjoy throughout the week.

SERVES 6

4–5 sweet potatoes (any kind)

METHOD 1:

1.  Preheat the oven to 375°F.

2.  Using a fork, perforate the skin all around each potato. This will help steam release while it is roasting.

3.  Arrange on a roasting pan or baking sheet and roast in the oven for roughly 45 minutes. When a fork slides through effortlessly, it's done!

4.  Store in the fridge for later use throughout the week.

METHOD 2:

1.  Preheat the oven to 375°F.

2.  Slice sweet potatoes thinly. Coat with coconut oil or butter.

3.  Roast in oven for roughly 20 minutes and enjoy!

# Sweet Potato Home Fries

This is a *great* brunch dish. People love sweet potatoes. It's a fact. A fantastic way to prepare this dish is to cook some bacon first, and then cook the sweet potatoes in the bacon fat. Then you can sprinkle the bacon on afterward. It's really lovely.

SERVES 2–4

1 or 2 large purple or white sweet potatoes, cut in ¼-inch cubes

1–2 tablespoons coconut oil or butter

pinch of salt

pinch of ground cinnamon

1. Place a large saucepan over medium heat. Fill it halfway with water.

2. Place the sweet potatoes in the water, and cover with a lid. Simmer sweet potatoes for roughly 7 minutes, or until a fork can almost slide easily through. Don't overcook!

3. Strain sweet potatoes and set aside.

4. Place a large skillet over medium heat. Wait until the pan is warm, and then add coconut oil or butter.

5. Add the sweet potatoes, stirring occasionally to brown the sides, roughly 4 minutes.

6. Add a pinch of salt and cinnamon and serve!

# Sweet Potato Mash

||||||||||||||||||||||||||||||||||||||||||||||||||||||||||||||||||||||||||||||||||||||||||||||||

SERVES 2

1 large baked sweet potato

¼ cup coconut milk or filtered water

¹⁄₁₆ teaspoon sea salt

¹⁄₁₆ teaspoon ground cinnamon

1. Place baked sweet potato in a medium saucepan, and using a fork, mash thoroughly with the coconut milk or filtered water.

2. Add the sea salt and the cinnamon.

3. Taste and adjust accordingly.

4. Serve with bacon bits, mixed with veggies, or with your favorite protein.

# Baked Portobellos

||||||||||||||||||||||||||||||||||||||||||||||||||||||||||||||||||||||||||||||||||||||||||||||||||||||||||||||

Mushrooms are pretty incredible. They are full of that umami flavor and are meaty and satisfying. Whenever I make polenta, baked portobellos are usually on the week's meal plan. Portobello mushrooms are in the same button mushroom family as white and crimini mushrooms. Portobellos are actually overgrown criminis! They are an excellent source of minerals and B vitamins and just a juicy, delicious addition to any meal.

SERVES 2

1 large portobello mushroom, cut in ¼-inch slices

1 tablespoon tamari

1 tablespoon extra virgin olive oil

1 tablespoon mirin

1.  Preheat oven to 375°F.

2.  In a shallow bowl, marinate the mushroom slices in the tamari, olive oil, and mirin. Coat each piece completely.

3.  Arrange the mushrooms on a large baking sheet lined with parchment paper or a glass baking dish.

4.  Bake for roughly 25–30 minutes, checking intermittently for doneness.

5.  Enjoy with shrimp and polenta, or Slow-Cooked Pork Ribs (page 165).

# Entrees

These next dishes hold meals together. They provide a nice shot of fats and proteins, and are full of flavor. They are meant to be added to a plateful of veggies and savored slowly.

Most of these recipes are designed to make in large batches so that you can bring some to lunch, and also freeze some for later.

# Sausage Lentil Broccoli Soup

||||||||||||||||||||||||||||||||||||||||||||||||||||||||||||||||||||||||||||||||||||||||||||

Lentils, compared to beans, are quick and make a tasty side dish or soup. They are a wonderful source of fiber, minerals, and protein. You could make this exact same recipe without blending, and it would also be delicious.

**SERVES 12**

2 cups green lentils

6 cups liquid (water or veggie/ bone broth; you can mix and match)

3 cloves garlic

2 bay leaves

1 large yellow onion, sliced

1 teaspoon ghee or coconut oil

1 head broccoli, roughly chopped

1 teaspoon ground cumin

¼ teaspoon turmeric

2 teaspoons sea salt

2 cooked sausages, sliced

salt and pepper, to taste

1. Add the lentils to a medium stockpot.

2. Pour in the liquid. The more broth in the total liquid you use, the more flavorful it will be.

3. Bring to a boil, and then simmer with the garlic and bay leaves for roughly 40 minutes.

4. In a separate sauté pan, sauté the onion until translucent in the ghee or coconut oil. Add to lentils.

5. Add broccoli to the pot and let it cook until you can stick a fork through easily.

6. Add cumin, turmeric, and sea salt.

7. Remove the bay leaves. Then, using an immersion blender, roughly blend the soup to the desired consistency. I like it slightly chunky.

8. Add the sausages and let simmer for 10 minutes.

9. Add salt and pepper, to taste.

10. Serve!

# Homestyle Black Beans

||||||||||||||||||||||||||||||||||||||||||||||||||||||||||||||||||||||||||||||||||||||||||||||||||||||

For a boost of protein and fiber, add beans to your scrambled eggs in the morning, or eat over rice topped with cilantro and avocado. Plus they are the perfect side dish to batch cook and freeze. I get excited when I remember I have beans in the freezer!

Organic canned beans are also great to use if you are short on time. Just check the label for added sodium and look for BPA-free cans.

MAKES ROUGHLY 3 QUARTS

2 cups soaked and drained black beans

1–2 quarts bone broth, veggie broth, or water

filtered water

3 bay leaves

1 large strip of kombu (optional)

1 large yellow onion, chopped

4 cloves garlic, chopped

2 tablespoons ground cumin

1 cinnamon stick

sea salt

1. Place beans and broth in a large stockpot or slow cooker.

2. Cover the beans with filtered water and add bay leaves and kombu, if using. If you are using a stockpot, cover and bring to a simmer for 1–2 hours. If you are using a slow cooker, cook overnight on low.

3. Sauté the onion and garlic in a medium sauté pan over medium heat. Add to beans. If you are using a stockpot, simmer for another 2–3 hours. If you are using a slow cooker, cook for another 6–8 hours.

4. Add the spices and salt, to taste. Cook longer if you want a more refried bean consistency. Freeze some, and enjoy the rest mixed with rice, greens, scrambled eggs, winter squash, or sweet potatoes!

||||||||||||||||||||||||||||||||||||||||||||||||||||||||||||||||||||||||||||||||||||||||||||||||||

**NOURISHING NOTE:** Whenever you cook beans, you should soak them the night before in roughly a tablespoon of baking soda. Beans like to soak in an alkaline medium to make them more digestible and less prone to making us gassy! Pour out the soaking water, and they are ready to use. The seaweed kombu is another addition that can help reduce gas, plus add nutrients. Do not cook beans with an acidic medium (lemon juice, tomatoes, or vinegar) as this will increase cook time.

||||||||||||||||||||||||||||||||||||||||||||||||||||||||||||||||||||||||||||||||||||||||||||||||||

# Coconut Red Lentils

Red lentils cook quickly and are highly nutritious. They are great for diabetics, as they have lots of soluble fiber and are a valuable source of folate, iron, and protein. I often make a large batch and freeze some so that on crazy weeks, I can pull a jar out of the freezer in a pinch.

SERVES 6–8

1 tablespoon coconut oil or butter

1 medium yellow or red onion, chopped

1 teaspoon turmeric

½ teaspoon mustard seeds

¼ teaspoon garam masala

2 teaspoons fresh minced ginger

2 cloves garlic, minced

2 cups red lentils

1 (13.5-ounce) can coconut milk

6–8 cups chicken broth or filtered water

sea salt and pepper, to taste

1. Place a large stockpot over medium heat. Add the coconut oil or butter.

2. Add onion, turmeric, mustard seeds, garam masala, ginger, and garlic, and sauté until onion is slightly translucent. Stir frequently.

3. When the onion is translucent, add lentils, coconut milk, and 6 cups of broth/water. Cover.

4. When lentils begin to simmer, turn heat to low and check, stirring periodically. They will burn quickly, so don't leave them alone too long.

5. If lentils become too dry, add more broth or water. Simmer for roughly 30 minutes, stirring frequently. Lentils are finished when they've reached a creamy consistency.

6. Add salt and pepper.

7. Eat some immediately, and freeze some for later use!

# Classic Seaweed Soup

||||||||||||||||||||||||||||||||||||||||||||||||||||||||||||||||||||||||||||||||||||||||||||||||||||||||||||||

This recipe is an adaptation of *miyukgook*, a Korean seaweed soup that's eaten for birthdays and is also given to nursing mothers. I taught this soup for a cooking class called "Nourishing Mamas" that I created with another chef and two pediatricians. We wanted to find a way to bring broth into the class and also teach a very simple and delicious soup. Bingo with this one. The seaweed is extremely mineral rich; it's a great source of calcium, iodine, and magnesium. Add any vegetables that you like, chopping them all to roughly the same size. The broth, seaweed, sesame oil, and soy sauce will add a distinct flavor.

MAKES ROUGHLY 3 QUARTS

2 big handfuls of kombu or wakame seaweed

1 cup filtered water

1 large pat butter or spoonful of coconut oil

2 large carrots, chopped

1 medium yellow onion, sliced

3 stalks celery, sliced

1 medium daikon radish, peeled and chopped

2 quarts beef broth

1 bunch of kale or collards, roughly chopped

sea salt or soy sauce and pepper, to taste

splash of toasted sesame oil

1. Taking a pair of scissors, cut kombu into ¼-inch pieces.

2. Place them into a bowl with 1 cup of filtered water. Set aside and soak for roughly 20 minutes.

3. Place a large stockpot over medium heat. Add the butter or spoonful of coconut oil.

4. Toss in soaked kombu and soaking water, carrots, onion, celery, and radish.

5. Stir on medium heat for roughly 5 minutes.

6. Add broth, cover, and simmer for roughly 45 minutes.

7. In the last 5 minutes, add in kale or collards.

8. Add salt or soy sauce and pepper, and a splash of sesame oil, and serve!

# Homestyle Ground Beef

I love ground meats. Pastured and organic meats can get expensive, so I recommend using ground meats since they are not only tasty and nutritious, but economical too. This dish is pretty darn versatile. You can make it more tomato-ey and use it as a pasta sauce, or mix it with rice, or have it over greens and an egg. You can also double the recipe and have it all week, and even freeze it. It's a great dish to batch cook.

When making ground meats over the stove, you can do it two ways. You can cook it until you don't see any more pink, and eat right away. However, I like to let ground meat simmer in the herbs and onions until it's tender and full of flavor. The proteins in meat will relax initially, but then tighten again. Longer cooking will allow the proteins to relax and become tender. If you aren't sure what tender tastes like, taste the meat as you go along, and you'll find the right consistency for you!

SERVES 4

1 tablespoon butter

1 medium yellow onion, chopped

1 pound grass-fed ground beef

½ (24-ounce) can stewed tomatoes

2 tablespoons minced fresh thyme

2 tablespoons minced sage

½ cup minced fresh parsley

1 cup bone broth or filtered water

1. Heat large a sauté pan until warm over medium heat, then add the butter.

2. Sauté the onion in the butter until translucent.

3. Add the ground beef, breaking up large bits and stirring occasionally.

4. Once the pink color has disappeared, add the stewed tomatoes, thyme, and sage.

5. Add the bone broth or filtered water.

6. Simmer on low with a lid, stirring occasionally for about 40 minutes or until beef is tender and soft. Garnish with fresh parsley and serve with brown rice, sauerkraut, and yogurt.

# Peanut Oxtail Stew

||||||||||||||||||||||||||||||||||||||||||||||||||||||||||||||||||||||||||||||||||||||||||||||||||||||||

Unlike the name suggests, oxtail is not from an ox! It's the vertebrae of the cow, and it's a fabulous, nutrient-dense part of the animal that makes a wonderful, gelatinous broth. Many different cultures have oxtail dishes, from curries to stews. This recipe is based off of a stew my mother made me and a Filipino dish called *kare kare*, which adds peanut butter for extra depth. It's also inspired by African cuisines that use peanuts (called groundnuts) and sweet potato in many soups and stews. Here, the sweet potato is roasted separately then added to retain its sweet flavor. This is one of my favorite things to make, so enjoy!

MAKES 3–4 QUARTS

2 pounds oxtail

2–3 quarts filtered water

1 tablespoon apple cider vinegar

1 large yellow onion, sliced

2 bay leaves

3 large carrots, chopped

1 (8-ounce) can of tomatoes (no salt added)

½ head cabbage, sliced

1 large sweet potato (preferably white fleshed), cubed

3 tablespoons peanut butter

cilantro sprigs, to garnish

1. In a slow cooker or stockpot, place the oxtail, and cover with the filtered water.

2. Add the apple cider vinegar and let simmer 8 hours or overnight.

3. Add the sliced onion, bay leaves, chopped carrots, tomatoes, and sliced cabbage. Let sit for another 4 hours in the slow cooker or simmer for another hour on the stove.

4. Preheat the oven to 375°F.

5. Using a fork, poke the sweet potato with superficial holes and roast for roughly 45 minutes. Remove from the oven when you can stick a fork clean through.

6. In a small bowl, ladle out a cup of broth, and add the peanut butter; stir until the peanut butter has dissolved. Add to stew.

7. Before serving, add in the cubed sweet potato and some minced sprigs of cilantro for garnish and color.

# Comforting Russian Borscht

The first time I made this soup, I was working on a farm on the central coast of California and one of my roommates was a Russian girl named Liz. Although she had spent much of her childhood in the Bay Area, she still had a strong connection with her Russian roots. I'm forever grateful to her for helping me adapt this simple recipe that I still make every winter. Beets are extremely nutrient rich, and their beautiful magenta color is a sign of that, although you could use golden beets as well. Beets are full of minerals, are great for the liver, and add a natural sweetness that most palates enjoy. It's hard to mess this one up!

SERVES 8

1–2 pounds beef shank or short ribs

1 teaspoon apple cider vinegar

1 pat butter or beef tallow (optional)

1 medium yellow onion, sliced

2 medium potatoes, chopped

2 cups sliced cabbage

4 medium beets, chopped

4 carrots, chopped

½ 24-ounce jar stewed tomatoes

sea salt and black pepper, to taste

For the optional garnish:
(mixed together or separate)

½ cup minced parsley

½ cup green onions

½ cup yogurt or sour cream

½ cup sauerkraut

1. If using a slow cooker, before going to bed, place the beef shank or short ribs in the slow cooker and cover with water. Add apple cider vinegar. Turn on low. If using the stovetop, place the beef shank or short ribs in a large stockpot and cover with water. Cover with a lid and simmer for about 1 hour.

2. Add onion, potatoes, cabbage, beets, carrots, and tomatoes straight into stockpot or slow cooker.

3. If using a slow cooker, set it on low for at least 4–6 hours and you are free to leave the house!

4. If using a stockpot, simmer on low for roughly 50 minutes. When a fork goes through beets easily, it's done!

5. Add salt and pepper.

6. Serve with parsley, green onions, yogurt or sour cream and sauerkraut, if using. Mix the garnishes together or use them separately, as desired.

# The Perfect Steak or Lamb Chop

Sometimes, I just feel like steak. For years, chefs have proclaimed that the best way to cook a steak is to sear the outside first, and then place it in the oven to finish cooking. A newer technique has come out recently to cook first in the oven, and then sear both sides quickly on the stovetop before eating!

You could go to a restaurant and have someone make it for you, or you could cook one up yourself *and* have some left over for dishes throughout the week.

SERVES 1–2

1 (5- to 6-ounce) sirloin or lamb blade chop steak

salt and pepper, to taste

1 tablespoon butter

1. Preheat oven to 375°F.

2. Season both sides of the steak with salt and pepper.

3. Place steak onto a large ovenproof pan on top of the butter.

4. Place pan into oven and cook for 7–8 minutes for medium.

5. Remove steak, and sear both sides for 1–2 minutes on high heat until each side is light brown on the outside.

6. Remove from heat and serve. I love to add more butter to my steak as I'm eating it...try it!

# Roasted Rosemary Chicken Legs

I was well into my late twenties when I discovered that you could use the oven to cook things. Gasp! In general, Asian cooking does not use an oven, and although my mother roasted chickens from time to time, we generally did not use the oven as much as we could have.

Now that I cook a host of things, the oven and kitchen timer are my dear friends. What a simple way to cook! You just stick it in the oven, set a time, and when you take it out, it's done! This recipe is exactly that. Plus, you can save the fat that runs into the bottom of the pan for cooking veggies later in the week.

SERVES 3–4

3–4 whole pastured or organic chicken legs

dash of sea salt

dash of chopped fresh rosemary

dash of chopped fresh thyme

1. Preheat the oven to 375°F.

2. Season both sides of the chicken with salt.

3. Optional: Heat a sauté pan on high. Add the chicken, and sear, cooking each side for about a minute until brown.

4. If you are using a cast-iron pan, you can leave chicken in the pan; otherwise, transfer the chicken to a piece of parchment paper on a baking sheet or a glass casserole dish.

5. Sprinkle with the rosemary and thyme.

6. Roast in the oven for about 45 minutes. When the juices run clear, it's ready.

7. Don't forget to save the bones for broth.

# Stewed Chicken

||||||||||||||||||||||||||||||||||||||||||||||||||||||||||||||||||||||||||||||||||||||||||||

This dish is a great way to use leftover chicken, and it's super versatile. You can put pretty much anything in, the base is just some yummy tomatoes and onions. Some nice ideas are coconut milk, mushrooms, quinoa, garlic, or kale.

SERVES 2–3

1 tablespoon coconut oil

1 medium yellow onion, sliced

1 (8-ounce) can (unsalted) or 2 fresh medium tomatoes, chopped

2 cups pulled chicken

splash of broth

sea salt and pepper, to taste

1. Heat a sauté pan over medium until warm.

2. Add coconut oil.

3. Add onion, stirring frequently until it is translucent.

4. Add the tomatoes.

5. Add the chicken and broth. Let simmer for 10 minutes.

6. Add salt and pepper.

# Chicken Curry Collard Wraps

Collard greens are an excellent whole food substitute for bread or tortillas to wrap up your ingredients. Plus, you can put anything in these, so it's fun to experiment. You can use collard wraps raw or blanch them to make them a bit more digestible.

This recipe assumes you're using leftover chicken, perhaps some Roasted Rosemary Chicken Legs (page 157) or roast chicken.

SERVES 1

1 teaspoon curry powder

½ cup whole plain yogurt

⅛ teaspoon sea salt

2 large collard leaves, stems removed

1 cup leftover roasted chicken

1 tablespoon raisins

¼ cup grated carrots

salt and pepper, to taste

1. Fill a medium pot with tap water and bring to a boil on high.

2. In a small bowl, mix the curry powder, yogurt, and salt together.

3. Add the chicken, raisins, and grated carrots.

4. Taste, and add salt and pepper as needed.

5. Once the pot of water is boiling, add the collard leaves and cook for 20–30 seconds or until the color changes to a bright green. Remove from the pot and hold under cool, running water.

6. Spread the collard greens on a plate, and put the chicken salad inside. Roll like a burrito.

7. Enjoy!

# Taiwanese Corn Soup

||||||||||||||||||||||||||||||||||||||||||||||||||||||||||||||||||||||||||||||||||||||||||||||||||

I remember my mother making me corn soup as a child. Corn is a delightfully sweet and comforting food, and the flavor that it adds to this simple soup is amazing.

This dish makes a wonderful first course or small snack, since it provides some quick nourishment to continue on with a busy day. It's much tastier using fresh corn, but if using canned, rinse the kernels to take off any added salt or sugar before adding it to the soup.

SERVES 2–3

1 quart chicken broth

1 can or 1–2 ears corn

¼ cup coconut milk

1 egg

salt and pepper, to taste

1. Heat the chicken broth in a medium saucepan over medium heat and add the corn.

2. If you are using fresh corn, let it simmer for a few minutes. If using canned, simply simmer for 1 minute.

3. Add the coconut milk.

4. Remove the soup from the heat and drop in the egg. Stir immediately. The egg should wisp into thin strips.

5. Season with salt and pepper. Serve and enjoy!

# Vermicelli Noodle Soup

I grew up eating noodles. They are quick and satisfying, but due to my nutrient-density mind-set, I've eaten less of them in my adult life. However, I still have vermicelli (bean thread) noodles around for when I need something quick and find my pantry to be a little bare.

SERVES 2

| | |
|---|---|
| 1 quart chicken broth | 2 eggs |
| 2 fist-size chunks of vermicelli noodles | 1½ cups roughly cut spinach or bok choy |

1. Fill one medium saucepan halfway with water and set to boil.

2. Fill another medium saucepan with broth and also set to boil.

3. When the water starts to boil, add the vermicelli noodles. (Or, you could always cook more and keep them in the fridge for more noodle soup or a stir-fry!) Boil for 2–3 minutes.

4. Taste for doneness. They should break apart easily, but not be mushy. Drain the noodles and set aside.

5. When the broth starts to boil, add the greens and simmer for 1–2 minutes.

6. Crack open the eggs and add them to the broth. Cover and turn off the heat.

7. Serve in bowls, one egg per serving, and add the desired amount of noodles.

# Chicken Miso Soup

This dish is inspired by my mother's home cooking and eating lots and lots of daikon radish growing up. Daikon is delightfully light and comforting, especially when it's cooked in soups. It's also considered to be detoxifying, anti-inflammatory, and full of nutrients. The recipe below is simply a guide, but include whatever you want, and add more miso if you want it saltier!

SERVES 4

1 medium daikon radish, chopped in 1-inch cubes

1 medium yellow onion, sliced

1 cup chopped shiitake mushrooms

2 quarts chicken broth

1 cup pulled chicken meat from leftover chicken (optional)

1 handful dried wakame

2 tablespoons miso paste, plus more to taste

1.   Place daikon radish, onion, and mushrooms into a medium stockpot with the broth.

2.   Simmer for roughly 30–40 minutes, until daikon cubes are translucent and a fork goes easily through them.

3.   Add the pulled chicken shreds, if using, and the dried wakame.

4.   In a small cup, ladle out ½ cup of the heated broth, and add the miso paste. Stir until dissolved and add into soup. Taste. Continue to add extra miso until desired taste is acquired.

# Kabocha Squash and Coconut Soup

||||||||||||||||||||||||||||||||||||||||||||||||||||||||||||||||||||||||||||||||||||||||||||||||||||||||||

This is one of my favorite soups. Winter squash by itself is such a treat, but there's something about the coconut and squash combo that is so satisfying. This recipe uses uncooked squash, but if you have leftover cooked squash, it's even quicker to make. You can use any squash, but kabocha is one of my favorites. You can even mix different kinds together.

SERVES 3–4

1 medium green, orange, or gray kabocha squash, cubed (can be substituted with 2 large sweet potatoes)

1 tablespoon butter or coconut oil

1 medium yellow onion, sliced

½ teaspoon ginger, minced

1 quart chicken broth

¾ cup coconut milk

sea salt, to taste

cilantro or pumpkin seeds, to garnish

1.  Add the kabocha cubes with 1 inch of water to a large pot and heat over medium. Cover.

2.  When the water starts to steam, turn down the heat and cook for 10 minutes or until you can easily stick a fork through the kabocha cubes.

3.  Heat a sauté pan on medium.

4.  Place the coconut oil or butter in the pan and add the onion and minced ginger. Sauté for 4–5 minutes, or until the onions are translucent.

5.  Once the kabocha is finished, add the onions, ginger, chicken broth, and coconut milk.

6.  Transfer to an immersion blender, and blend until smooth.

7.  Return to the pot and simmer for another 10 minutes. Add filtered water or coconut milk if you desire a more liquid consistency.

8.  Add salt. Serve with cilantro or pumpkin seeds.

# Taiwanese Tacos

When I go back to Taiwan, pork is everywhere. I find it delicious, versatile, and comforting. The recipe below is basically the way you make most ground pork dishes, including the filling that you put in dumplings and in buns. I use this as a guide to make meatballs, or I just make a meat sauce that I use throughout the week. This recipe is great for a brunch, and the lettuce wraps give it a beautiful crunch and clean taste. The pork can also be eaten over rice, stuffed in half a delicata squash, or in a veggie stir-fry.

SERVES 3–4

1 pound pastured ground pork

¾ cup water or bone broth

½ medium yellow onion, chopped

½ cup chopped mushrooms (optional)

2 tablespoons soy sauce (tamari if going gluten free)

1 teaspoon sesame oil

2 tablespoons rice wine or mirin (optional)

3 cloves garlic, minced

½ teaspoon ginger (optional)

1 head romaine lettuce, separated

1. Place the ground pork in a large, lidded sauté pan over medium heat. Using a fork, separate the pieces until the entire pan is covered. Add the water or bone broth and stir occasionally.

2. Add the onion and mushrooms to the pan and stir in the tamari or soy sauce, sesame oil, and the rice wine or mirin, if using.

3. Add the garlic and ginger, if using, and mix with the pork. Cover with a lid.

4. Lower heat to medium-low and let ground pork simmer for approximately 20–30 minutes, stirring occasionally. Keep adding water or bone broth to make sure pork is simmering in liquid.

5. Occasionally taste pork until meat is tender and when ready, remove from heat.

6. Plate with a few lettuce leaves and make little tacos immediately before eating! Enjoy!

# Slow-Cooked Pork Ribs

This dish is a reason to love your slow cooker. You literally put the ingredients in and come home to lovely smells. I tend to finish the ribs off, and then have some great broth with which to cook veggies in or make a little stew afterward. Enjoy!

SERVES 3–4

2 pounds pork ribs

3–4 cups filtered water or pork broth

5–6 crimini or shiitake mushrooms, sliced

1 cinnamon stick

2 star anise

1 small yellow onion, sliced

3 garlic cloves, chopped

2 large (roughly thumb-size) slices ginger

2 tablespoons tamari sauce

1 tablespoon mirin rice wine

½ teaspoon apple cider vinegar

sea salt and pepper, to taste

1. Slice each pork rib individually and place into the slow cooker.

2. Using the broth or filtered water, barely cover the ribs.

3. Add the rest of the ingredients, except the salt and pepper.

4. Cook on low for 6–10 hours.

5. Add salt and pepper.

6. Eat over rice and with a side of greens.

# Miso-Glazed Dover Sole

||||||||||||||||||||||||||||||||||||||||||||||||||||||||||||||||||||||||||||||||||||||||||||||||||||||||||||||||||||||||

I love cooking fish because it's so darn quick. If you need to throw something together for dinner, this dish is something that takes minimal effort and packs a great amount of flavor. Plus, Dover sole is on the Monterey Bay Aquarium Seafood Watch list of sustainable seafood!

SERVES 4

1 pound Dover sole, sliced

2 tablespoons white miso

2 tablespoons filtered water

lemon juice (optional)

1. Preheat oven to 350°F. Line a cookie sheet or baking pan with parchment.

2. In a small bowl, mix the miso and water together until blended. Pour onto a small plate.

3. Coat fish slices with the miso mixture on both side, and place on the cooking sheet. Transfer to oven.

4. Bake thin slices for 6–7 minutes; thicker slices for 8–9 minutes. If you have mixed thicknesses, you may want to remove slices that are thinner when they are done.

5. Garnish with fresh lemon juice, if desired, and serve with a grain and a veggie!

# Lemon Salmon

Salmon is one of the easiest things to make and is extremely high in omega-3 fatty acids, which are essential for brain function and heart health. It's also extremely high in selenium, which is important for prostate health and thyroid function.

Wild Alaskan salmon is the salmon of choice. It's sustainable and is the least contaminated among fish in general. If you cannot find fresh or frozen Alaskan salmon, canned salmon is the next best choice.

**SERVES 2**

1 (6- to 8-inch) salmon fillet

dash of sea salt

fresh or dry rosemary sprigs (optional)

lemon slices (optional)

1. Preheat oven to 375°F.

2. Sprinkle both sides of the salmon fillet with salt.

3. Place the salmon fillet on a baking pan. Add rosemary or lemon slices, if using, on top.

4. Bake for roughly 10 minutes and check. You can use a fork to see if pieces flake off. It's okay if the salmon is slightly rare in the middle.

5. Remove from oven and let rest for 5 minutes. Garnish with lemon additional lemon slices and serve!

# Salmon Stew

IIIIIIIIIIIIIIIIIIIIIIIIIIIIIIIIIIIIIIIIIIIIIIIIIIIIIIIIIIIIIIIIIIIIIIIIIIIIIIIIIIIIIIIIIIIIIIIIIII

This recipe was another recipe we used in our Nourished Mamas cooking series. It has few ingredients and is incredibly delicious. The heartiness of the potatoes goes well with the lightness of the salmon.

Oftentimes, a great way to make fish broth is to buy fish heads at the store. Usually discarded, fish heads are actually a powerhouse of nutrition—they're full of iodine, which is necessary for thyroid health. Remember that fish broth only needs a short simmering, 20–30 minutes and done!

SERVES 4

1 tablespoon butter or coconut oil

2 medium yellow onions or leeks

3 cups water, chicken broth, fish broth

¾ pound potatoes, cubed

1 bay leaf

¾ cup cream or coconut milk

¾ pound salmon filet, skinned, de-boned, and cut into small chunks

salt and pepper, to taste

fresh parsley or dill, to garnish

1. Heat a large stockpot over medium heat until warm.

2. Add the butter or coconut oil and throw in sliced leeks or onions.

3. Sauté until translucent. Add broth or water.

4. Add cubed potatoes and bay leaf, and let simmer for 15 minutes until soft.

5. Add cream or coconut milk, and then add fish.

6. Simmer for another 5 minutes.

7. Add salt and pepper.

8. Throw in parsley or dill and turn off heat. Serve.

# Garlic Shrimp

||||||||||||||||||||||||||||||||||||||||||||||||||||||||||||||||||||||||||||||||||||||||||||||||||||||||||||

Shrimp! I am a big fan. It reminds me of being home with my mother. Plus, it's another one of those quick-to-make dishes. According to the Seafood Watch, you should avoid shrimp from Mexico. Nutrition-wise, shrimp is packed full of selenium (which we need for healthy thyroid function), protein, and vitamin B12.

You can buy shrimp with the heads on, or peeled and deveined. If you buy with the heads, you can cook without shelling, then shell them at the table, which is super fun. You can also buy with shells and no heads. In this case, I like to shell them and use a knife to slice the back and pull out the vein. It's strangely satisfying.

SERVES 3–4

1 pound shrimp, peeled and deveined

2 tablespoons soy sauce

2 tablespoons mirin

½ teaspoon toasted sesame oil

1 tablespoon coconut oil

2 cloves garlic, minced

1. Marinate the peeled shrimp in a medium bowl with the soy sauce, mirin, and sesame oil. Mix these ingredients thoroughly and marinate in the fridge for at least an hour. Heat a medium sauté pan over medium and coat the pan with coconut oil.

2. Add shrimp, marinade, and minced garlic. Let cook for about a minute and stir occasionally.

3. Cook until the shrimp is a nice, pink color.

4. Serve over polenta, congee, rice, or quinoa!

# Sweet Treats

My clients and I do a lot of work to get refined sugar out of the diet. The goal, however, is not to cut out sweets entirely. There are wonderful options to indulge in that come from whole foods and that are simple and quick to make. The following recipes are great to bring to parties because they are a beautiful way of introducing healthy sweet treats to friends and family. Enjoy!

# Avocado Chocolate Mousse

You can make delicious things from avocados. This "whoa" dish is one of them. Avocados are high in potassium, vitamin E, B vitamins, and healthy fats. This dish is a sure crowd pleaser, especially with the avocado surprise factor! You can serve it with seasonal fruit, and the presentation looks amazing.

SERVES 4

| | |
|---|---|
| 3 avocados | ¼ cup maple syrup |
| 4 pitted dates | 1 teaspoon ground cinnamon |
| 2–3 tablespoons cocoa powder | ¼ teaspoon sea salt |
| ½ cup coconut milk | |

1. Using a spoon, scoop the avocado out into a large mixing bowl or the food processor.

2. Add the dates, cocoa powder, coconut milk, maple syrup, cinnamon, and sea salt.

3. Using an immersion blender or food processor, blend all of the ingredients together until smooth.

4. Taste. Add more of any ingredient if necessary.

5. Serve on its own, as a dipping sauce for fruit, or as an icing for cake!

# Zucchini Bread

||||||||||||||||||||||||||||||||||||||||||||||||||||||||||||||||||||||||||||||||||||||||||||||||||||

My mother used to make the best zucchini bread. Zucchini is amazing because it adds delicious moisture to baked goods, and it's a way to sneak in some veggies! This recipe is a gluten-free version using coconut flour and very little added sweetener.

**MAKES 1 LOAF**

1 cup raisins

2 tablespoons coconut oil, divided

1 ripe banana

1 heaping tablespoon almond butter

1 teaspoon vanilla

2 tablespoons maple syrup

4 eggs

1 teaspoon baking powder

1 teaspoon baking soda

½ cup coconut flour

½ teaspoon salt

1 teaspoon ground cinnamon

1/16 teaspoon ground nutmeg

2 cups shredded zucchini

1. Soak the raisins in a bowl with water. Set aside.

2. Preheat the oven to 375°F.

3. Use half of the coconut oil to grease a loaf pan. You can also cover the bottom with parchment paper that comes up the sides of the loaf pan. This makes for easy removal.

4. In a large bowl, place wet ingredients: banana, remaining coconut oil, almond butter, vanilla, maple syrup, and eggs.

5. Using a whisk, mixer, or immersion blender, mix until smooth.

6. Add the dry ingredients: baking powder and soda, coconut flour, salt, cinnamon, and nutmeg. Mix until smooth.

7. Add the zucchini and drained raisins and fold in until evenly distributed.

8. Pour into loaf pan.

9. Bake for 45–50 minutes. Check periodically; center should not look wet.

10. Allow to cool, slice, and enjoy!

# Fudge Bumpkins

These make great after-dinner treats or quick snacks on the go. Plus, most kids love them, and if you wanted, you could sneak some more goodness into them, like chia seeds, kelp, or spirulina and chlorella. I sometimes make these as parting gifts when I throw events, or I use the same recipe and make bigger bars to take with me. Use cashews, pecans, macadamia nuts, almonds, or the nuts of your choice. You can add anything to these, so experiment!

**MAKES 16 BUMPKINS**

1 cup raw, unsalted nuts

1½ cups pitted Medjool dates

2 tablespoons ground flaxseeds

¼ cup shredded, unsweetened coconut

2 tablespoons unsweetened cocoa powder

1 teaspoon vanilla

½–1 tablespoon melted coconut oil

¼ cup ground cinnamon, cocoa powder, and/or coconut shreds, for dipping

1.   Blend nuts and dates in food processor or using a large bowl and an immersion blender until well combined.

2.   Add all of other ingredients except the oil and dipping ingredients. Blend again.

3.   Test consistency. It should be sticky and hold together. If it is dry, add some melted coconut oil until the dough sticks together.

4.   Roll dough into small balls. You can roll the balls in coconut flakes or cocoa powder or cinnamon for a beautiful coating.

5.   Enjoy immediately or refrigerate for several days.

# Coconut Chia Seed Pudding

||||||||||||||||||||||||||||||||||||||||||||||||||||||||||||||||||||||||||||||||||||||||||||||||||||||||||||||||||||||

I was obsessed with eating this pudding when I first discovered it. The creaminess of the coconut milk was just so satisfying. Plus, since I had been scared of fat all my life, this little treat was what taught me that I can enjoy it and not worry about putting on weight. Coconuts themselves are amazing, and I use them often in my cooking. They are rich in manganese, molybdenum, copper, selenium, and zinc. Much of the fat in coconuts are medium-chain fatty acids, which the body converts most readily into fuel.

This pudding is great as a snack, with seasonal fruit, or with the addition of cocoa for a little extra fun. Put it in a jar to take with you during the day. Once you open a can of coconut milk, store the leftover in a jar and put it in the fridge. It will stay good for around 4 days; smell it before using it!

SERVES 1

| | |
|---|---|
| 1 tablespoon chia seeds | ½ teaspoon maple syrup |
| ¼ cup filtered water | ⅓ cup coconut milk |

1. Soak chia seeds in water for 10–15 minutes.

2. Add maple syrup to chia seed mixture after soaking.

3. Add coconut milk, stir, and enjoy!

# Summary Fruit and Mint Yogurt Lassi

Lassis are a traditional yogurt drink from India. At restaurants, they're frequently prepared with mango, and are usually very, very sweet. I like this version because it uses the natural sweetness of ripe summer fruits, adds a bit of mint, and has a nice tangy taste from the yogurt. The lime adds another beautiful dimension. Try this on hot summer day, and share with friends.

SERVES 4

2 cups seedless watermelon or 1 large, ripe peach

¼ cup lightly packed mint

1 cup whole milk plain yogurt

¹⁄₁₆ teaspoon (roughly a pinch) salt

juice of 1 lime

sprig of mint, to garnish

1. Place all of the ingredients in a blender. Blend and serve with a sprig of mint!

# Cashew Milk Shake

Cashews are simply amazing because of their *creaminess*. The texture of soaked cashews with a little filtered water is just heavenly, especially if you are like me and try to avoid dairy as much as possible. Cashew cream is super yummy and can replace regular cream. Plus, nutrient-dense cashews are higher in protein and carbohydrate than other nuts. That said, feel free to add nutrient boosters, such as spirulina or flax—great for kids.

MAKES ROUGHLY 3 CUPS

1 cup cashews, soaked for at least 1 hour and drained

2 cups filtered water

2 tablespoons cocoa powder

2 pitted Medjool dates

⅛ teaspoon ground cinnamon

⅛ teaspoon vanilla

⅛ teaspoon sea salt

1. Place all of the ingredients in a blender.

2. Blend and serve.

# Date Almond Milk

**MAKES 1 QUART**

1 cup overnight-soaked almonds

4 cups filtered water

2 pitted dates

¼ teaspoon vanilla

¹⁄₁₆ teaspoon sea salt

½ teaspoon ground cinnamon

1. Place soaked almonds and water in a blender and blend.

2. Using a clean dish towel or finely meshed sieve, strain into a separate container.

3. Set aside almond pulp for use in pancakes or baking.

4. Rinse blender, and place strained almond milk back into blender with dates, vanilla, sea salt, and cinnamon.

5. Taste and adjust seasonings.

6. Enjoy immediately, or store in fridge for 3–4 days.

# Mexican Hot Chocolate

Plain cocoa powder is full of antioxidants and oh so rich and satisfying. This is something that I use to treat myself on a cold winter day.

SERVES 1

1 cup filtered water, almond milk, or coconut milk

1 tablespoon cocoa powder

pinch of ground cinnamon

pinch of cayenne pepper

pinch of sea salt

1 teaspoon maple syrup

1. Heat water or milk in a small saucepan over a low flame.

2. When warm, add cocoa powder, cinnamon, cayenne, sea salt, and maple syrup.

3. Taste. Add more of any ingredient as desired.

# Holistic Nutrition 101

So far in this book, we talked about a holistic overview of health, and then a detailed guide to nourishing yourself for 21 days with the Nourished Belly Diet. This next section is for those of you that want to learn more about nutrition, and *why* the Nourished Belly Diet is the way it is. I personally think it's important information for all of us to learn, but I'm also into this level of detail...so read on if you want to find out more!

It's funny that we eat every day, and yet, the average person gets little nutrition education. The information we do receive is always focused on what we should avoid, and fruits and vegetables. The education should be centered around what the body needs to function at its prime. That said, let's do a quick Nutrition 101 tutorial.

Basically, your body needs two things: energy and building blocks for body structures. Some things, your body has the ability to make on its own (especially if you are healthy), but others you must get through the food you eat. So you need to eat.

Let's talk about energy first. The body is incredible. The amount of things that have to happen as soon as you bite into something for it to be delivered to your cells is astounding. Essentially, you are looking for glucose, a sugar that will feed your cells directly. Where do you get glucose? You get it from carbohydrates, which is one of the three macronutrients that you need larger amounts of in your diet.

Carbohydrates come from vegetables, fruits, starches, and sugars. Depending on the form they come in, they could be complex, with lots of molecules bound together, or they could be simple, with a very simple molecule chain. This is where you might also hear the terms poly-, oligo-, di-, or monosaccharides. The prefixes of these words refer to the number of simple sugars bound together. The body, though, has to transform these more complex sugars into simple sugars to absorb them and convert everything into glucose, which is used by the body for energy.

When you eat simple sugars, like candy, you absorb it rather quickly, which is not something you want. You want to absorb things slowly over time. When you eat an excess of simple carbohydrates, your bloodstream is flooded with glucose, so your fat tissues store it as fat.

The fat that you store in your body is different from the fat you eat in foods, which is different from the fat that is part of your bodily structures. Confusing! Let's first look at the fat you eat, which is the second macronutrient that you need in larger amounts.

Dietary fat is taken in by the body and broken down into its parts. One glycerol molecule and three fatty acid molecules. Together these are called triglycerides—sound familiar? Fatty acid molecules can be described by length as short-, medium-, or long-chain fatty acids. They can also be described as either saturated or unsaturated. Whether or not a fatty acid is saturated or unsaturated depends on the number of hydrogen atoms bonded to the core carbon atoms. Saturated fatty acids are full of hydrogen atoms, while unsaturated are missing either one hydrogen atom (monounsaturated) or more than one (polyunsaturated). We've all heard these terms before, but they are very rarely explained.

For all intents and purposes, foods are filled with a variety of all of these different types of fatty acids, and you should eat a bit of all of them.

The broken-down glycerol and fatty acids enter the liver and your fat cells. In the fat cells, they are put back together into triglycerides and stored for later. When there is a lack of glucose, the body then breaks down triglycerides to be used as energy in the form of fatty acids. You are constantly switching between glucose metabolism and fat metabolism throughout the day.

Fat is also used within the body to make up certain structures. Each cell membrane is created from layers of fat. Cholesterol is also a type of fat that you can get through food, but your body makes a majority of it. Cholesterol is a building block for hormones, such as estrogen and progesterone, and is part of the tissue that surrounds each nerve.

Proteins are the final macronutrient, and they also serve as building blocks that you need to maintain your bodily structures. Over "100,000 different proteins are thought to exist in the body."[40] Proteins are made up of different combinations of amino acids, and there are roughly 20 naturally occurring amino acids, 12 of which your body can make as long as you are in good health, and eight other amino acids you must get from food—these are called essential amino acids. You can also use protein as energy, but it is not the preferred energy source.

You need three macronutrients: fat, protein, and carbohydrate. You also need nutrients called *micro*nutrients. These are the vitamins and minerals that you probably have heard a lot about. The Institute of Medicine created Daily Recommended Intakes (DRIs), which are the levels recommended to a healthy population to prevent disease. (I personally don't like to get too bogged down with numbers and instead choose to focus on eating a variety of foods, which is what this book is all about!)

---

40 Kapit, Wynn, Robert I. Macey, and Esmail Meisami. *The Physiology Coloring Book.* 2nd ed. San Francisco: Addison Wesley Longman, 2000.

Vitamins and minerals are responsible for chemical reactions in the body; they are usually paired with an enzyme to either build up or break down components in the body.

Vitamins are broken up into two types: fat soluble and water soluble. Fat-soluble vitamins can be stored in fat cells and used when needed. They include:

- Vitamin A
- Vitamin D
- Vitamin E
- Vitamin K

Water-soluble vitamins can only be stored in small amounts, so deficiencies can develop more easily. They include:

- Thiamine (B1)
- Riboflavin (B2)
- Niacin (B3)
- Pantothenic acid (B5)
- Pyridoxine (B6)
- Folic acid
- Vitamin B12
- Biotin
- Choline
- Vitamin C

Each of these vitamins serve specific functions in the body; oftentimes, it took diseases to help us understand what exactly they did. Scurvy, discovered on long sea voyages, where gums and joint capsules bleed and wounds fail to heal, was caused by a vitamin C deficiency. Beriberi, documented first in Asian countries, caused numbness, and eventually, paralysis, was discovered to be a thiamine deficiency.

Minerals are also broken up into two categories: major minerals and minor minerals. We need more than 100 mg daily of these major minerals.

- Calcium
- Chloride
- Magnesium
- Phosphorus
- Potassium
- Sodium
- Sulfur

Following are minor minerals, also called trace minerals:

- Boron
- Chromium
- Copper
- Iodine
- Iron
- Manganese
- Molybdenum
- Selenium
- Silicon
- Vanadium
- Zinc

Minerals are absorbed with adequate stomach acid, and plants are mineral rich if the soil they are grown in is mineral rich. This is another reason to buy from farms whose priority it is to enrich the soil, which small organic farms aim to do.

# Bioavailability

One more thing to discuss while we are on the topic of nutrition: bioavailability. Bioavailability is the body's ability to absorb nutrients from the foods we eat. We've all heard, "You are what you eat." It's true, but one of my favorite sayings in nutrition school at Bauman College was: "You are what you can absorb." Before going to school, this was never something that even crossed my mind. We have to absorb stuff? The health of your digestive system is very much influenced by what and how you eat. Let's talk about ways to maximize absorption.

RULE 1: Chew! Think about food being broken down into smaller particles, which have more surface area for your saliva or your stomach acid to break down. The smaller bits are also easier for your intestines to continue breaking down, so you absorb more.

RULE 2: Always eat carbohydrates with a bit of fat. Many carbohydrates, such as fruits and vegetables, have amazing vitamins and minerals, some of which are fat-soluble. Therefore, eating your greens coated with a bit of healthy fat will enhance absorption. This goes for smoothies and juices too—add a bit of coconut milk or flax oil to enhance digestion.

**RULE 3:** Check your stomach acid. You need adequate stomach acid to break apart your minerals and to absorb vitamin B12 in your intestines. This vitamin needs to be brought down there by binding with something called the intrinsic factor. You only have good amounts of intrinsic factor if you have adequate stomach acid.

To do a quick home stomach acid test, first thing in the morning, drink 1 cup water, with 1 tablespoon of baking soda mixed in. You should let out an enormous belch within the next five minutes. If you don't, then that could be a sign that your stomach acid levels are low. A great way to start to remedy this is to drink a ½ cup of water with 2 teaspoons of apple cider vinegar before meals.

||||||||||||||||||||||||||||||||||||||||||||||||||||||||||||||||||||||||||||||||||||||||||||||||||||||||||||

**NOURISHING NOTE:** Supplements can be a tricky subject. Many, many people ask about which supplements they should take. I personally tend to stay away from taking too many supplements unless I'm sick or recovering from an injury.

Things to think about:

- Some forms of supplements are more absorbable than others. For example, iron citrate is a more absorbable form of iron than sulfate or fumarate.

- Look for high-quality supplement brands (reputable brands include Standard Process, Designs for Health, Thorne, Metagenics, Innate Response, Nordic Naturals, Carlsons, New Chapter, and Garden of Life, to name a few).

- Check with your health-care provider if you have health issues; even supplements can interfere with your course of treatment.

||||||||||||||||||||||||||||||||||||||||||||||||||||||||||||||||||||||||||||||||||||||||||||||||||||||||||||

**RULE 4:** Eat *everything you can.* Variety here is key, and it doesn't matter if you are vegan, vegetarian, pescatarian, carnivore.... Certain nutrients need other nutrients for absorption, like vitamin

D is necessary for calcium absorption,[41] magnesium is necessary for calcium absorption, zinc and copper need to be in balance, potassium and sodium, etc. The list goes on and on.

# Tips for Healthy, Nourishing Cooking

Cooking is a skill; it's not something that can purely be taught through a book. It has to be experienced: You burn things, oversalt dishes, and overcook steaks, and then you force yourself to eat what you cook 'cause you spent some cash on those ingredients!

Recipes, like the ones in this book, are merely guides. They can lead you to a great-tasting meal, but depending on your ingredients or how hot your stove is, you have to be engaged in the process of cooking. Checking things, tasting things…it's an art form.

One of my favorite books is *The Flavor Bible* by Karen Page and Andrew Dornenburg, precisely because I don't like to follow recipes. I love this book because it tells you what flavors go together. So when I happen to have a piece of lamb at my house and don't want to run to the store, I will look in the book and see what flavors go well with lamb that I already have in my pantry. I also love their review of the four flavors: bitter, salty, sweet, and sour. Learning to cook starts with experimenting on how to balance these flavors.

There is also a fifth flavor that the Japanese call umami. Umami is a mouthfeel, and what we also call savory. We now know that this is due to an amino acid called glutamate, and it is why so many processed foods add monosodium *glutamate* (MSG)—to enhance the flavor of their snacks. Glutamate naturally occurs in mushrooms, Parmesan and blue cheese, tomatoes, anchovies, soy sauce, miso, and walnuts. It makes sense that these ingredients are in so many dishes!

---

41 "Calcium," Micronutrient Information Center, accessed September 15, 2015, http://lpi .oregonstate.edu/mic/minerals/calcium.

Learning how to cook at home is really learning how to taste and know what could be missing. In the beginning, it can be a challenge just to experiment with salt. Salt can be tricky, because too much can make a dish inedible (well, you can always add more ingredients or broth to lessen the saltiness), but just the right amount of salt brings out all the right flavors. Not to mention that everyone's salt preference is different. Start by adding one-eighth teaspoon, stir, taste, add a pinch more, and taste. Get acquainted with the taste that you like! Then you can start experimenting with lemons and adding sauerkraut, different oils, and spices.

# Cooked Versus Raw

Another question that people often ask me is whether or not they should eat foods cooked or raw. Raw food enthusiasts say that there are enzymes in raw foods that are destroyed with heat, and it's true that enzymes are destroyed at 118°F. However, traditional Chinese medicine and Ayurvedic nutrition wisdom both support eating cooked food.

There are pretty opposing nutritional philosophies out there, and certain people might do really well following one.

Again, I'm a moderate, and from what I know from both science and what makes sense to me, you can do a mix of things.

Some nutrients are heat sensitive; vitamin C and pantothenic acid, for instance, degrade with heat. Others, like lycopene, are enhanced through heat. Cooking will break open cell walls, which makes the nutrients more available to us!

I also love how both traditional Chinese medicine and Ayurveda describe the stomach as a simmering pot and your digestive fire. When you eat foods cold and uncooked, you lower the temperature of your simmering pot, just like when you bring a pot up to a simmer and add an ingredient, then need to wait for it to come to a boil again. Your digestion is much the same way. So according to these traditional ways of looking at nutrition, eating cooked foods and warm foods is better for your digestion.

I personally subscribe to eating cooked, warm foods, unless it's summertime, when I feel like eating more salads. Same goes for drinking warm liquids or room-temperature liquids. It's really hard to for me to drink ice water, unless it's after an intense workout or it's super-hot outside.

I judge what's good for me on how I feel after eating. I feel really, really good when I eat a warm, delicious stew. This, again, is going to be different for everyone. I also eat things raw on occasion, definitely more in warmer months and especially when I'm snacking on something.

Eat a mixture, then. If you have primarily uncooked raw foods, eat cooked foods once in a while. If you have mainly cooked foods, do some raw food snacks.

Find a balance that you feel good with.

# Quick Cooking Tips

- Start with fresh ingredients. This is probably the *most* important. There is nothing you can do to a sad tomato to make it taste good.

- Know the source of your ingredients. This matters for both quality and taste.

- Practice cutting with a knife. Protect your fingers by tucking them in, and make round surfaces flat. That way, you aren't in danger of something rolling while you are cutting it.

- Add whole spices to soups and braises to help blend flavors. They release flavor more slowly, since they are whole.

- Add powdered and crushed spices at the end so that their aroma and flavor don't fade by the time you serve.

- Don't be afraid of cooking oil! You want to coat a heated pan, and you want to coat the food.

# Where Do You Go from Here?

Congratulations! Hopefully, you've experimented with some form of the Nourished Belly Diet, and whatever has happened, you undoubtedly have learned something! Whether it be something about your own habits, or learning to make something new in the kitchen, you've taken steps forward in creating better health.

So, now what? Where do you go from here? The purpose of this book is to start looking at food as a wonderful way to take care of the amazing body you have. Continue to use the Weekly Planner, and work on one thing each week or every couple of weeks. Reflect on what works for you and what doesn't. Remember to take some time outs to reflect and remember that YOU are ultimately responsible for your own health.

Thank you for taking the time to give back to yourself. It's been a wonderful experience putting these thoughts down on paper, and I hope that you've been able to get something from it!

With love,

Tammy

# Appendix A:
## Guide to Healthy Cooking Oil

I often get asked which cooking oils are healthy to use at home. First of all, oils matter. They coat the dish, spread the flavor, and can be healthful or harmful. You want to think about how much processing it takes to extract the oil, if the plants are genetically altered, and how you plan on cooking. Here are a few oils that I suggest for cooking.

**COCONUT OIL:** Coconut oil is great for increasing metabolism. The body loves to use it as energy. It's made of primarily short- and medium-chain fatty acids. Coconuts have a lot of great properties. As an oil, it's stable to cook with and adds a lovely flavor. I also use it for oil pulling and moisturizing.

**OLIVE OIL:** Olive oil is a monounsaturated fat and is great for adding flavor. I often drizzle it on soups and veggies, and sometimes use it for cooking when I know I'm not frying anything.

**AVOCADO OIL:** Avocado oil is another monounsaturated fat that has a milder flavor. Some people prefer to cook with avocado oil instead of coconut oil for this reason.

**GHEE:** Ghee is clarified butter, which means all the protein solids have been taken out, and it is pure fat. It's expensive to buy at the store, but super simple to make at home. (You'll find the recipe on page 100.) I think it smells like a fresh, buttered croissant and gives your dishes this aroma! One of my favorite dishes is mushrooms cooked in ghee—heavenly! If you are going to fry anything, ghee is a great choice since it has an extremely high melting point.

**ANIMAL FATS:** Chicken schmaltz, beef tallow, pork lard—these were all once vilified, but are now making a comeback. Animal fats (from healthy, organic animals of course), are great to cook with and add amazing flavors. I often skim the fat off my bone broths and save these in the fridge to cook with.

---

What about canola, grapeseed, and peanut? I often get asked about these oils, since most of them are advertised as heart healthy and safe for cooking over high heat. These oils tend to be high in omega-6 fatty acids. Canola, for example, is pretty much all genetically altered. I tend to stay away. Toasted sesame oil is an ingredient that I usually add to the end of cooking for flavor.

# Appendix B:
## Guide to Antioxidants

Ever wondered exactly what antioxidants were in what? This short guide will give you a quick overview of what you get when you eat your colors.

## Betaines

These compounds are water soluble, sensitive to heat and light, and responsible for the bright pinks and yellows in a few fruits and vegetables. Betaine functions closely with other compounds that act as "methyl donors." These compounds donate a methyl molecule in the key process called methylation, which ensures proper liver function, cellular replication, and detoxification. Methylation also helps your body synthesize brain chemicals. It helps control homocysteine (which can damage blood vessels) and is important in detoxification. Betaine has the ability to help the liver process fats and could lessen the damaging effects of alcohol on the liver.

Food sources of betaine include beets, chard, fish, legumes, amaranth, and the prickly pear.

## Chlorophyll

Chlorophyll is the green pigment in plant cells, where light is converted into sugars. Each chlorophyll molecule has one magnesium atom centered in the middle. From whole foods, chlorophyll is fat soluble; thus, you should cook them with a fat for better absorption. Fat-soluble chlorophyll can stimulate hemoglobin and red blood cell production. Chlorophyll supplements, on the other hand, are mostly water soluble and are not absorbed from the gastrointestinal tract. They are used to sooth the GI tract and reduce fecal odor. Natural sources include green leafy vegetables, broccoli, wheat grass, and algae.

# Flavonoids

Flavonoids, or bioflavonoids, are a large family of phytonutrients synthesized in plants. They lend the vibrant red, purple, blue, white, and yellow colors to many fruits, veggies, and flowers. They include many compounds, some of the better known ones being anthocyanins and anthoxanthins. Flavonoids are sometimes called vitamin P and serve as antioxidants in the body, fighting a broad range of oxidants. Flavonoids have powerful anti-inflammatory, antiviral, antiallergic, and anticancer properties.

ANTHOCYANINS: Anthocyanins are in the flavonoid family and appear red, purple, or blue depending on the pH. They serve many functions in plants, including signaling and protection from pathogens. In the human body, these colors increase the vitamin C level within our cells, decrease the leakiness of blood vessels, and help prevent the destruction of collagen (important for healthy skin and tissue). Anthocyanins are found in grapes, berries, apples, red cabbages, and red potatoes.

Anthoxanthins range from white to more yellow in acidic conditions. Anthoxanthins exert general antioxidant activity and support the immune system. They are found in citrus fruit, onions, cauliflower, potatoes, turnips, and garlic.

# Carotenoids

First found in carrots, this large family of chemicals includes over 600 compounds. Some of the better known are beta carotene, xanthophyll, and lycopene. They are fat soluble, so are better absorbed when cooked with fat, and retain their bright yellow, orange, and red colors when cooked.

Carotenoids are found in two different places in plants: in cells that determine color, and together with chlorophyll. Carotenoids protect chlorophyll from damage, acting as antioxidants for the plants by neutralizing the harmful by-products of photosynthesis (conversion of sunlight to energy in a plant cell). They also act as antioxidants in the human body. Some of the carotenoids are considered pre-vitamin A compounds, meaning they are converted to vitamin A in the body.

Studies show that the consumption of naturally occurring carotenoids help protect against skin, lung, uterine, and cervical cancers, heart disease, cataracts, and other degenerative diseases caused by oxidative stress.

*Beta carotene* was the first carotenoid to be discovered and is perhaps the best known, but is only one of many antioxidant carotenes with pre-vitamin A activity. These carotenes are converted into vitamin A in the body. Beta-, alpha-, and gama-carotenes are the predominant pigments in orange foods such as carrots, winter squash, apricots, mangos, and yams. *Lycopene* is a carotenoid that studies have shown reduces the risk of several types of cancer. Lycopene is responsible for the bright pinks and reds found in tomatoes, watermelon, pink grapefruit, apricots, pink guava, salmon, and paprika. *Xanthophyll* is a group of carotenes that include compounds such as lutein. It is one of the primary divisions of the carotenoid group and supplies the vivid yellow to the family. Foods high in xanthophyll are yellow squash, corn, pineapple, turmeric, ginger, saffron, egg yolk, and yellow bell pepper.

# Appendix C:

## Complete List of Belly Boosters

### Algae

Algae are single-celled, photosynthetic organisms that grow in freshwater lakes and ponds. We'll talk about two specific types of algae: spirulina and chlorella. Both contain bioavailable essential fatty acids, chlorophyll, active enzymes, vitamins, minerals, complex sugars, and phytonutrients and help with heavy-metal detox.

**SPIRULINA (BLUE-GREEN ALGAE):** Spirulina grows naturally in lakes that have a high acidity. It is free-forming and floats on the surface of the water. One of the most primitive forms of plant life, spirulina was used by the Aztecs and some Africans as an important food staple. Spirulina is up to 77 percent a complete and readily digestible protein. It is cooling and detoxifying and supports all organ functions. It lowers cholesterol, enhances the immune system, and is also cancer protective. It is also helpful for the digestion by increasing beneficial bacteria.

**CHLORELLA:** The first plant to grow with a true nucleus, chlorella has been on earth for more than 2.5 billion years. It's a superior source of assimilable chlorophyll, which helps to cleanse and detoxify cells in the body (a clean and healthy cell can better utilize other nutrients). Chlorella is helpful for chronic gastritis, high blood pressure, diabetes, constipation, anemia, and high cholesterol. Chlorella is similar to spirulina, but has less protein and more chlorophyll. It contains all essential amino and fatty acids and is very rich in lysine. One teaspoon has 6 grams of protein!

||||||||||||||||||||||||||||||||||||||||||||||||||||||||||||||||||||||||||||||||||||||||||||||||||||||

**NOURISHING NOTE:** Alone, these algae have intense flavors, so they work well mixed in with something sweet or something salty.

||||||||||||||||||||||||||||||||||||||||||||||||||||||||||||||||||||||||||||||||||||||||||||||||||||||

# Herbs and Spices

Herbs and spices are a delicious and easy way to expand your culinary talents, as well as increase the amount of nutrients you are putting into your body. This is the one area that *everyone* can grow in because so many cultures have different flavor profiles. It's an ever-evolving way to connect to other people and to expand on what you can make at home. I'm always learning some new spice to add to my own cooking.

Fresh herbs keep for a week or so in the fridge. Dried herbs can often be more potent, so you need less of them in cooking. Dried herbs also lose flavor and nutrients over time, so no need to buy in bulk unless you are planning on using a lot of it within a year. Going through and changing out old herbs is a good idea.

Here are some great herbs and spices to start with, and expand from here.

CAYENNE: A pinch of cayenne can help to increase metabolism, is great for colds and flus—and can help as a digestive aid. Even those that don't like spices can appreciate a pinch of cayenne in their hot chocolate; you'll find this in the Mexican Hot Chocolate recipe on page 178.

CUMIN: I use a lot of cumin; for me, it was the gateway drug of spices. Cumin comes from the parsley family and is beneficial to the liver and digestion. *The Flavor Bible* advises to add it early in cooking, and if you are using the seeds, to toast them in a dry pan before using them. Cumin goes great in beans, hummus, and lentils.

GARLIC: A powerhouse, garlic is known as a folk remedy for knocking out colds. It not only adds a ton of flavor, but is also antifungal, antibacterial, and antiviral. It is a staple in Asian cooking that I add liberally to most veggie stir-fries. Raw garlic is much more pungent than cooked, so be mindful if you have a date!

**GINGER:** Ginger is great for winter months, as it helps to warm the body and increase metabolism. It's becoming most well-known for its anti-inflammatory properties and helping to settle an upset stomach. If you aren't all about eating it, you can add a few large chunks to soups and stews that you fish out later.

**SEA SALT:** Salt in your food isn't the enemy. Sodium and potassium work closely together and serve an important function in the body: bringing nutrients into a cell, and bringing waste out through the sodium-potassium pump.

However, in the Standard American Diet (SAD), we take in too much sodium and too little potassium. Around 75 percent of our sodium comes from packaged foods and restaurants,[42] while only 6 percent of our salt intake comes from the salt shaker.[43]

If you are a generally healthy person, be wary of how much processed foods you consume and how much eating out you are doing, but at home, salt your food to taste. I stay away from table salt, because it fits into *Pandora's Lunchbox* author Melanie Warner's definition of a processed food: You can't make it at home. Table salt is refined, and chemicals are added to keep it from caking and bleached. Any trace minerals are refined away. Sea salt, on the other hand, is literally just salt from evaporated sea water; plus, it's got lots of minerals in trace amounts (which we just need a little of each day). And, there are different colors to experiment with and add to your dish: black, red, pink, to name a few.

**ONIONS:** Onions are an extremely nutrient dense and fantastic food! Slow cook them to release the sugars to sweeten any meal, and get a fantastic dose of antioxidants. They are versatile enough to go with almost any meal.

---

42 Brody, Jane. "Sodium-Saturated Diet Is a Threat for All." *New York Times*, December 26, 2011, http://www.nytimes.com/2011/12/27/health/high-sodium-to-potassium-ratio-in-diet-is-a-major-heart-risk.html?_r=0.

43 Moss, Michael. *Salt, Sugar, Fat: How the Food Giants Hooked Us.* New York: Random House, 2013.

**PEPPERMINT:** Peppermint is great on a hot summer day; it helps to cool the body. It is also great with digestion, helpful for relaxing muscles, and extremely high in antioxidants. Mint is great to garnish salads and adds a wonderful flavor to dishes. I use it in my Cilantro Mint Hummus on page 106 and in the Summer Fruit and Mint Yogurt Lassi on page 175. Peppermint is not advised for those who suffer from heartburn or gastroesophageal reflux disease (GERD), since it can relax the esophageal valve.

**ROSEMARY:** Rosemary grows in almost every corner of California. You can use it in baked goods, on potatoes, or with baked meats. Rosemary is an adaptogen, which means that it helps the body deal with stress, as well as being excellent for memory and high in antioxidants.

**THYME:** Thyme is great in stews and soups, as well as being a powerful herb. It's high in antioxidants and has antimicrobial and antifungal properties.

**TURMERIC:** Turmeric's beautiful color is a great sign of antioxidants. Turmeric is becoming very well-known for its compound called curcumin, recognized for its anti-inflammatory properties. Turmeric is often combined in Indian dishes with coriander and cumin. You can buy powdered or fresh turmeric and grate it directly into dishes.

## Nuts and Seeds

Nuts and seeds are a great addition to lots of different dishes and will add a crunch that is a trick to making a dish really enjoyable. They are also great sources of proteins and fats, and make really great snacks, as well as belly boosters. Below are some suggestions of great nuts and seeds to add to your pantry collection of belly boosters. Most nuts and seeds should be stored in cool dark place, but to be on the safe side, as many nuts and seeds have very delicate oils that are susceptible to spoilage, can be stored in the freezer or fridge, and used immediately.

**BRAZIL NUTS:** I didn't always eat Brazil nuts. They were always the last ones left in the nut mix. Am I right? It's only after going to nutrition school that I've started adding them into my nut rotation. One interesting fact about these nuts is that they come from trees that don't like to be tamed, so most trees remain wild in the Amazon Valley in Brazil, Peru, and Bolivia. Brazil nut pods fall from a height of about eight stories, and collectors wear shields to protect themselves from falling pods! I'm always amazed at information like this, especially because at times we can balk at the price of highly nutritious food at stores. So, knowing how difficult it is to collect something makes me understand that the price reflects the hard work put into cultivating and harvesting.

Brazil nuts are prized mainly for their selenium content; selenium is a key nutrient in metabolism. It is also part of the antioxidant glutathione, it works with vitamin E to prevent free radical damage.[44] Brazil nuts are great in nut mixes and crushed and added to oatmeal.

**CHIA SEEDS:** Chia seeds, after flaxseeds, have the highest source of plant-based omega-3 fatty acids in the form of alpha-linolenic acid. They also become very mucilaginous when soaked and can relieve constipation and soothe the intestines. The black and gray spotted chia seeds are nutritionally superior to the golden chia variety. Chia seeds can be substituted for poppy or sesame seeds as a garnish.

- Use chia seeds to make a refreshing drink. Hydrate 1 tablespoon of chia seeds in ½ cup of water and let soak for 10 minutes, stirring once or twice. Add preferred liquid (like coconut water, coconut milk, or juice) and enjoy! (Try Coconut Chia Seed Pudding on page 174)

- Instead of using cornstarch or flour, add ground chia seeds to thicken soups or gravies until you reach the desired consistency.

---

44 Murray, Michael T., and Joseph E. Pizzorno. *The Encyclopedia of Healing Foods.* New York: Atria Books, 2005.

- Add ground chia seeds to an egg, or with a little water, to bind together meatballs or hamburger patties.

- Using a sprouting kit or a mason jar with a cheesecloth and rubber band, rinse chia seeds, pour off excess water, and let sit. Every twelve hours, rinse with water and drain off excess. In two days, you should have little sprouts to add to salads.

**FLAXSEEDS:** Flax is a native Mediterranean plant that has been used for over 5,000 years. Flax is a good source of dietary fiber, magnesium, potassium, and manganese. It includes the essential omega-3 fatty acid alpha-linolenic acid (ALA) and phytoestrogens, also known as lignans. ALA can be converted into long-chain fatty acids such as EPA and DHA, but the conversion can be faulty in some individuals, especially those with diabetes and nutritional deficiencies. ALA by itself has been shown to reduce the risk of heart disease and cancer. Lignans can bind to estrogen receptors and interfere with cancer-promoting effects on breast tissue and also have antibacterial, antifungal, and antiviral properties.

Flax becomes very mucilaginous in water and can therefore be very soothing to the intestines and bowels. The tiny, flat brown seeds, rather than the golden variety, are a superior source of fatty acids. Whole, they can be stored at room temperature, but ground they quickly can go rancid in a week's time. It is better to grind them immediately before eating. Store flaxseed oil in the refrigerator.

Ground flax can be spread over oatmeal, granola, and cooked veggies; baked in breads; used in smoothies; or added to savory dishes.

**HEMP SEEDS:** I love to suggest hemp seeds to clients because they are extremely easy to add to any dish. Yes, the hemp plant is the same as the marijuana plant, but just like there are different types of tomatoes, there are different types of cannabis plants. You won't get to an altered state from eating hemp seeds, nor will you test positive in drug tests!

Nutritionally, hemp is a powerhouse. Hemp is a source of omega-3 fatty acids, and also gamma-linolenic acid (GLA), which is the type of omega-6 fatty acid that is anti-inflammatory. It's also a complete protein; I much prefer athletes use raw hemp seeds in smoothies instead of protein powders.

**PUMPKIN SEEDS:** Pumpkin seeds are not only yummy, but they are great on salads, in granolas, and as a garnish for soup. They are also a wonderful, cost-effective replacement for pine nuts in pesto. Healthwise, they can be used to supply nutrients for a healthy prostate, and are a great source of minerals. My mother soaks them with garlic and then dehydrates them in the oven for a nice flavor—go Mom!

## Seaweed

Sea vegetables are one of the most nutritious foods you could eat. Most famous in Asian cultures, they also are used in Irish cultures, among the Inuit, and other coastal peoples. They are incredibly mineral-rich, with the mineral content being 7 to 38 percent of their dry weight.

They help to reduce blood cholesterol, remove radioactive and metallic elements from the body, support the thyroid, counter obesity, strengthen bones, teeth, and nerve function, and help improve digestion. The most significant elements are calcium, iodine, phosphorus, sodium, and iron. Seaweed is also a rice protein source, containing up to 38 percent protein. It is also an above average source of vitamins A and B.

The easiest way to use seaweed is as a condiment and in soups. Any type can be sprinkled onto your stir-fries, mashed potatoes, salad, or popcorn. I add kombu or wakame to any bean, rice, or lentil dish and cook everything together. They are an extremely easy way to add nutrient density to your diet.

Whole seaweeds hold up really well in soups and stir-fries, while flaked seaweeds work great as a garnish. More well-known types are wakame, kombu, dulse, nori sheets, and arame, among many more. You'll find seaweed in the Sardine Nori Wraps (page 104) and the Classic Seaweed Soup (page 151) in the recipe section.

## Zest

Zest is the top layer of citrus fruits. It contains essential oils that can brighten up any dish, not to mention that the compound limonene in zest is great for liver detoxification. I most commonly use the zest of lemons, oranges, and limes. You can either use a Microplane to grate, or using a vegetable peeler or knife, slice off the outermost layer, and slice into smaller chunks.

# Appendix D:

## Protein in Common Foods

(per 3.5 oz or 100 grams)

| Meats | |
|---|---|
| Red meat | 23.4 g |
| Pork loin | 27.57 g |
| Turkey | 26.59 g |
| Chicken | 23.97 g |
| Lamb | 24.52 g |
| **Fish and Seafood** | |
| Cod | 17.9 g |
| Halibut | 26.69 g |
| Mahi mahi | 23.72 g |
| Salmon | 19.94 g |
| Shrimp | 20.91 g |
| Tuna | 29.91 g |
| Crab | 19.35 g |
| Shellfish | 6–7 g |
| **Cheese and Dairy** | |
| Cheddar | 24.9 g |
| Cow's milk | 3.29 g |
| Yogurt | 5.25 g |
| Feta | 4 g |
| Cream cheese | 2 g |
| Ricotta (½ cup) | 14 g |
| Cottage cheese (½ cup) | 14 g |
| Milk (1 cup) | 8 g |
| Most hard cheeses | 6–7 g |
| Yogurt (1 cup) | 12 g |

| Eggs (1 whole egg) | |
| --- | --- |
| Whole | 6.2 g |
| Whites | 3.5 g |
| **Beans and Legumes** | |
| Black beans | 8.9 g |
| Chickpeas | 8.86 g |
| Kidney | 8.67 g |
| Lentils | 9.02 g |
| Mung | 7.02 g |
| Navy | 8.7 g |
| Pinto | 8.21 g |
| Tempeh | 18.54 g |
| **Veggies** | |
| Artichokes | 3.48 g |
| Asparagus | 2.58 g |
| Broccoli | 2.98 g |
| Brussels sprouts | 2.55 g |
| Cauliflower | 1.84 g |
| Kale | 3.3 g |
| Spinach | 2.86 g |
| **Nuts (per 1 oz/roughly one handful)** | |
| Almonds | 3 g |
| Brazil nuts | 2 g |
| Cashews | 2 g |
| Chestnuts | .45 g |
| Hazelnuts | 2.1 g |
| Flaxseed | 2.8 g |
| Macadamia nuts | 1.1 g |
| Peanuts | 3.4 g |
| Pecans | 1.31 g |

Taken from Michael Murray's *Encyclopedia of Healing Foods*

# Appendix E:
## Tea It Up!

After going to nutrition school, one of the changes in my kitchen was an entire cupboard dedicated to herbal teas. They all inhabit cute little mason jars, and I've created a label for each. It's adorable.

Teas are a wonderful and delicious way to enhance what you put into your body every day. The recommendations below are based on what I learned at nutrition school and also from friends and colleagues who are herbalists. These are the most common herbs that I introduce and recommend to my clients to add to their hydration rotation. Teas are a generally mild way to ingest an herb, but if you have any severe health issues, it's always good to check with your health provider if you have reservations.

**CHAMOMILE:** A member of the daisy family, chamomile is a soothing herb tea effective for nervousness, anxiety, stress, and insomnia. It strengthens the immune system, soothes the digestive tract, eases headaches and allergies, and supports the gall bladder. It can also be poured into your bath as a relaxing addition. Popularly drunk before bedtime, chamomile is also a source of health promoting flavonoids, vitamins, and minerals.

**DANDELION:** Dandelion is an extremely powerful herb. You can sauté and then eat the leaves, and the root is often made into a coffee substitute. You can also use both the leaves and root for making tea. The leaves alone can be bitter, so I often like to mix them with other teas, such as mint. Dandelion root tea has a strong, earthy flavor that coffee drinkers usually enjoy. The root is most well-known for aiding the liver, helping to increase bile production, and causing the release of stored bile in the gallbladder. Caution: Those who have gallstones or other bile duct obstructions should ask their doctor before using this herb.

**GINGER:** Second only to salt as an Asian condiment, Indian Ayurveda regards ginger as the "universal medicine." It has many healing properties and is a warming addition to any food. Studies show that ginger is an effective remedy for motion sickness and nausea, and is a potent anti-inflammatory. It is traditionally used to calm the digestive system and to strengthen the immune system. Fresh ginger is preferred, for it has higher levels of anti-inflammatory compounds, but ground ginger also has positive effects. Always look for plumpness and when buying more mature ginger; scraping the skin off with a spoon is especially effective. To make a tea, dice a few slices and simmer, or simply let steep for five to 10 minutes.

**HIBISCUS:** A brilliantly red-colored infusion, hibiscus (also called Jamaica) is a tangy, cranberry-like drink that is full of vitamin C and minerals. Studies show that drinking hibiscus tea can reduce hypertension. Due to its high vitamin C content, it is best brewed with room-temperature water to preserve vitamin content. Latin stores will often carry hibiscus; look for packages marked "flor de Jamaica."

**KUKICHA:** Kukicha is another mildly earthy tea that I love. Kukicha is the Japanese word for twig, and thus this tea is made from the twigs of the tea plant. (The same tea plant is used for green, black, oolong, pu-er, and white tea, just with different processing). This tea has the least amount of caffeine of all the tea plant teas and is a lovely addition to a meal.

**MINT:** Mint is a wonderful tea to introduce into your daily diet. It is delicious as an after-meal digestive, soothing your digestive system, especially your colon. Mint also helps disperse pathogens and promotes circulation. It can alleviate symptoms of mastitis, painful menstruation, and hives. Buy fresh mint when possible; the fresh leaves can also be used for salads or ground up in ice cream or smoothies. As a tea, it is a good source of manganese, vitamin C, folate, iron, magnesium and calcium. As a fresh leaf, it is also a source of carotenoids (including beta-carotene) and dietary fiber.

*Caution:* For those having painful menstrual cramps due to fibroids, cysts, or endometriosis, mint is not recommended. Do not use peppermint for infants; spearmint, on the other hand, may be used.

**NETTLES:** Nettles are the first tea that I introduce to clients. They are one of the more nutrient-dense teas and have a mild, grassy flavor that people tend to love. Nettles are a weed and are found all over the United States. They are also called stinging nettles because their stiff, bristly hairs found on the leaves and stems inject a stinging fluid into the skin. An interesting note is that the sting can be used therapeutically as a treatment for increasing circulation and arthritic conditions. However, the sting isn't pleasant, so if you find a patch to harvest, handle it with care! Heat and drying destroys the sting.

Nettles are extremely high in vitamins and minerals, including vitamin C, vitamin K, carotenes, and iron. You can let fresh or dry nettles steep all day, as all the water-soluble nutrients will leach out. The deep green is the chlorophyll, which is an excellent source of magnesium. For maximum absorption, drink the tea while eating a bit of fat. My fellow nutrition friend Corinne Steel uses a bit of flaxseed oil that she pours into her carrot juice to better absorb the carotenes. Same idea with chlorophyll; it has both fat and water-soluble components.

Fresh nettles can be sautéed like spinach and are delicious! Don't forget to add some butter for better absorption.

**RED RASPBERRY:** Red raspberry is full of nutrients, such as magnesium, B vitamins, and iron, but it is probably most well-known for helping during the menstrual cycle and pregnancy. It helps to tone the uterine wall and can be helpful in cramping, and possibly making the way for smoother births!

**ROOIBOS (ROY-BUS):** Native to the Western Cape of South Africa, this herb is sometimes served with milk as a tea latte. However, it is excellent by itself and a good substitute for black tea because it has a more robust and full flavor. It is caffeine-free and a great source of antioxidants, vitamin C, and minerals.[45] Traditional uses include alleviation of allergies, nervousness, asthma, skin problems, and digestive complaints. Brew for three to five minutes; it can be brewed multiple times without becoming bitter.

**TULSI:** Another stress-relieving tea, tulsi tea, also called holy basil, is in the same class of herbs as chamomile. They are both adaptogens; meaning they help the body adapt to stress. Tulsi also provides a healthy dose of vitamins, minerals, and antioxidants and is antifungal and antibacterial. This tea is *not* recommended for women trying to get pregnant.

---

45 Balick, Michael J., and Andrew Weil. *Rodale's 21st-century Herbal: A Practical Guide for Healthy Living Using Nature's Most Powerful Plants.* New York: Rodale, 2014.

# Recommended Resources

## Books

*Animal, Vegetable, Miracle* by Barbara Kingsolver

*The Encyclopedia of Healing Foods* by Michael T. Murray and Joseph Pizzorno

*Fat Chance* by Robert H. Lustig

*The Flavor Bible* by Karen Page and Andrew Dornenburg

*In Defense of Food* by Michael Pollan

*Lights Out* by T. S. Wiley and Bent Formby

*The New Whole Foods Encyclopedia* by Rebecca Wood

*Nourishing Traditions* by Sally Fallon

*The Omnivore's Dilemma* by Michael Pollan

*Real Food* by Nina Planck

*Salt, Sugar, Fat: How the Food Giants Hooked Us* by Michael Moss

*Why Zebras Don't Get Ulcers* by Robert M. Sapolsky

## Web Resources

Cornucopia Institute
www.cornucopia.org
The Cornucopia Institute is an educational group committed to organic and sustainable practices. A consumer watchdog for organics, the institute takes political action to safeguard clean eating and farming practices. They have a great scorecard of organic dairy and eggs!

### The Environmental Working Group (EWG)
www.ewg.org

This consumer watchdog and political action organization does its best to keep our food system clean by looking under the rug at products and foods that are available to the public. An excellent resource, their website includes the Dirty Dozen and Clean 15 Guides, sunscreen and body care ratings, and grocery product ratings.

### Fair Trade USA
fairtradeusa.org

Purchasing items with the Fair Trade Certified label is one of the ways that you can buy ethically. Farmers that are part of this organization are guaranteed a fair wage, and it usually applies to products that must be imported and cannot be grown in the US, like chocolate, bananas, coffee, and tea.

### Non-GMO project
www.nongmoproject.org

### Organic Resources
create.extension.org/sites/default/files/WhyEatOrganicBW2012
Handouts.pdf

### Seasonal Food Guide
www.sustainabletable.org/seasonalfoodguide

### The Story of Stuff
storyofstuff.org

This website and organization has *great* video resources on things that matter, such as what our consumerism does to the environment, what bottled water really is, and more. Perfect for teachers and parents who want to engage children in learning how to better the economy and environment.

### Weston A. Price Foundation
www.westonaprice.org

If you want to talk traditional foods, the Weston A. Price Foundation is *the* resource; their website has a lot of great information. You can become a member and receive a quarterly journal.

# Index

# Acknowledgments

This book would not have been possible without the support of my family, who perhaps with some hesitancy, have always supported me to follow my dreams. I thank my soul sisters and brothers, many of whom are in the healing and movements arts, who have always encouraged me to share my gifts with the world and have inspired me to keep learning and thriving. Thank you to Bauman College and the incredible teachers at the Berkeley location for providing me a wonderful foundation with which to spread health and happiness. Lastly, thank you to the capoeira community, without which the opportunity for this book would not have been possible, and for all the support you have given me throughout the past and many years to come.

# About the Author

Born in Ohio and raised by Taiwanese parents, **Tammy Chang** now finds her home in the Bay Area. In addition to her nutritional work with clients and groups, she teaches fitness and is the head instructor at a capoeira school in Oakland.

Before being certified in holistic nutrition by Bauman College, Tammy received a BA in public policy from Duke University, and as a New York City Teaching Fellow received her MA in childhood education from Brooklyn College.

In her free time, she loves to roam the California forests and hot springs, sample restaurants, watch or read the latest sci-fi series, practice handstands, and spend time with family and friends.